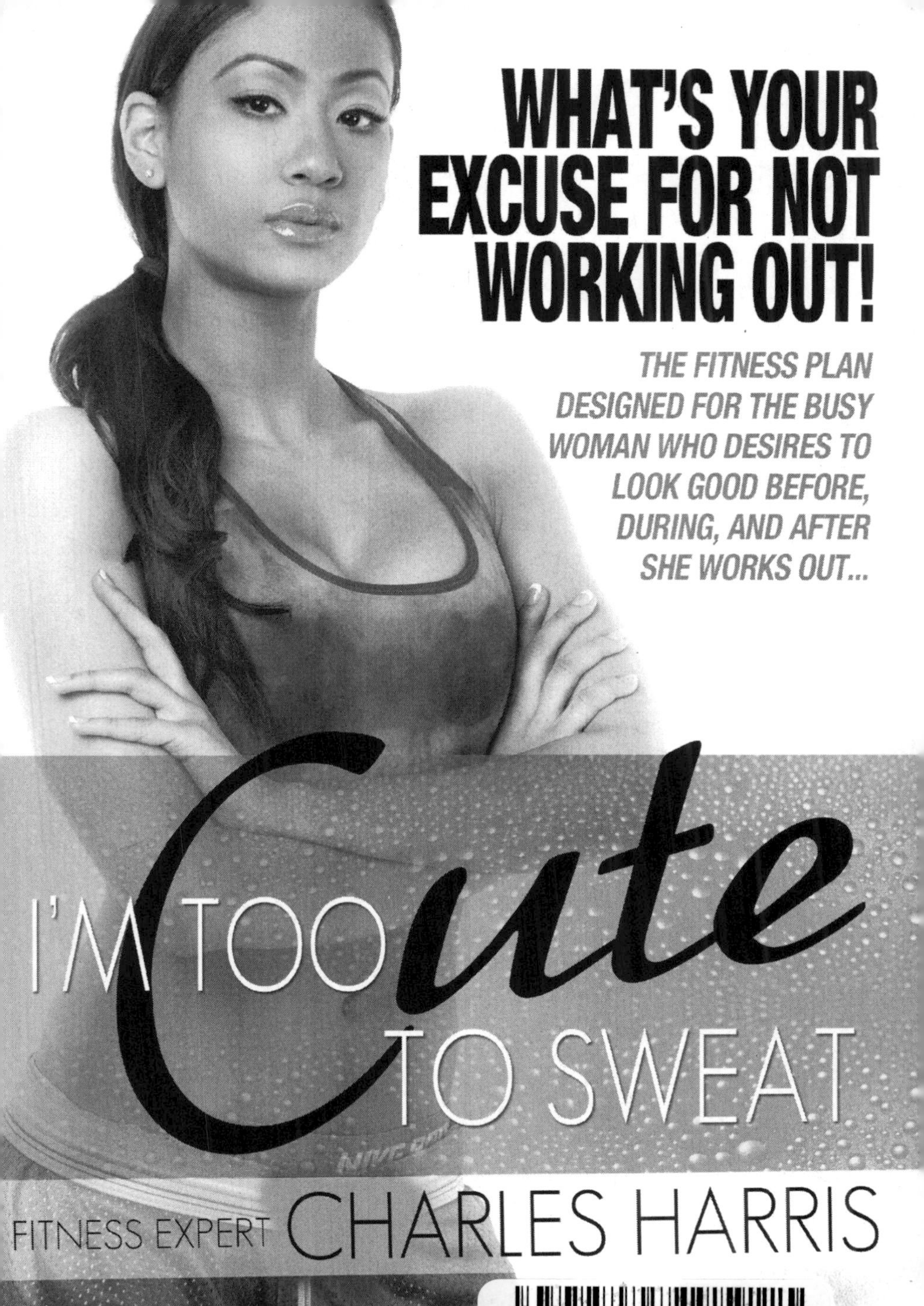
WHAT'S YOUR EXCUSE FOR NOT WORKING OUT!
THE FITNESS PLAN DESIGNED FOR THE BUSY WOMAN WHO DESIRES TO LOOK GOOD BEFORE, DURING, AND AFTER SHE WORKS OUT...
I'M TOO Cute TO SWEAT
FITNESS EXPERT CHARLES HARRIS

ISBN 13: 978-0-615-56289-6

Typesetting: Marion Designs
Editor: Finding Definition, LLC
I'm Too Cute To Sweat/by Charles Harris
For complete Library of Congress Copyright info visit;
www.chizelit.com

Liz You are a amazing woman! This is your year! 2012

Acknowledgments

Thank you, Lord, for using me as a vehicle to help enrich the lives of so many people over the years. I would like to honor my lovely wife of nineteen years, Donna, to whom this book is dedicated. She is truly the woman who has been there with me through thick and thin. Without her support, this book would not have been possible. She is my first and only love who means the world to me.

I would also like to thank my sweet mother Beatrice Harris for always being in my corner for encouragement and kind words. Thank you as well to my son Domeniq and daughter Charlesha.

I give special thanks to my Pastor Karen Bethea of *Set the Captives Free Outreach Center Baltimore, Md.*, to Sharon Page, author of *Eat Your Food Naked*, to Mia Redrick of *Finding Definitions LLC* and all of my clients who played a significant part in the creation of this book.

I love you all!

Contents —

Forward

I'm Too Cute To Sweat is a wonderful compilation of information that will challenge women to reconsider incorporating fitness into their busy lifestyles and routines. With an alarming rate of women stricken with heart disease and obesity, it would benefit us to become proactive in our approach to health. Some of us are so busy that we are literally falling apart. Why wait until we are falling apart and need to see a doctor before the thought of physical health crosses our mind? Thanks to this marvelous and generous work by fitness expert Charles Harris, women on the go can now find ways to include a workout into their schedules. I encourage each reader to take the 21 day challenge. It will literally transform the way you see yourself, life, and others. Utilize the tips that are located in each chapter. Jot down your plan. We have to write the vision and make it plain so that we can run with it and enjoy it.

As a pastor of a demanding congregation, I value the sessions that I have with Mr. Harris. Not only do I leave feeling rejuvenated, but I am able to relieve stress and stay fit. While I have to fit time for fitness into my schedule, I would not be able to maintain my schedule without it. You can't keep driving a car and never give it any maintenance. Nor can you keep working your body to the ground and never refurbish it. Exercise is the way to a lean, strong, and healthy body!

The best part about becoming fit is that it does not have to be expensive. There are things that you can do right at home, in the office, and in the car to keep your body operating at maximum efficiency. Take the time, you can't afford not to! I encourage you to read this book from cover to cover and discover how easy it will be to incorporate into your daily routine. Remember our bodies are the temple of the Lord. We will one day have to give account for how well we did or did not preserve it. The answer is now in your hands. Enjoy!

Dr. Karen Bethea, Senior Pastor
Set the Captives Free Outreach Center
Baltimore, Maryland

INTRODUCTION

"I'm Too Cute to Sweat" is a life changing book dedicated to women of all ethnicities. With the number of heart disease and obesity cases steadily increasing in America, women are being stricken at an alarming rate. When it comes to health and fitness, women usually fall into one of three categories. The first category is the workout junkie: She works out every day - or at least three days a week. The second is the weekend warrior who exercises only on weekends. The third is the majority of American women: They are just too busy to work out. However, they are usually very overweight and suffer from health problems; I call them the "Couch Potatoes!"

What I hope to do is build a bridge for those women; those who find it difficult to exercise because of their busy schedules or for other reasons beyond their control.

Contrary to popular belief, it *is* possible to maintain a busy life *and* still have time to live a healthy lifestyle - Physically, Mentally, and Spiritually. It will take some time management and a little sacrifice but together we will make it happen.

Too many women are dying today prematurely because of heart disease, stress, and obesity. I believe with a little "push" and a game plan, women who don't want to exercise or don't have time to take care of themselves can be rejuvenated and have a shift in mindset about the importance of living a healthy lifestyle. For over a decade, I have helped thousands of women reach their fitness goals— **and now I would like to help you!** This book is the key to help you overcome many of your excuses and challenges. Health and wellness is imperative for living a happy and productive life. No matter how spiritual you are, if you are not healthy it will be a hindrance to you and your happiness and the plan that God has for your life. Because women are nurturers by nature, they are designed to take care of so many other individuals before they take care of themselves. However I truly believe that self-preservation is the first law of nature.

I have been blessed with the gift of being able to encourage women to push beyond their barriers to achieve a healthier lifestyle. I've heard every excuse in the book for not working out hair, kids, career, spouse, or just plain laziness—but time and again, in the course of just one conversation, I have been able to find a plan that works for each individual's lifestyle. You will be amazed how in just 21 days you can transform your Mind, Body and Spirit in ways that you previously couldn't even imagine. I believe if you really embrace these simple techniques and principles, your life will never be the same. I look forward to helping you over the next 21 days to achieve all of your fitness goals, to live a healthier lifestyle and last but not least, I look forward to helping you create the body you have always desired!

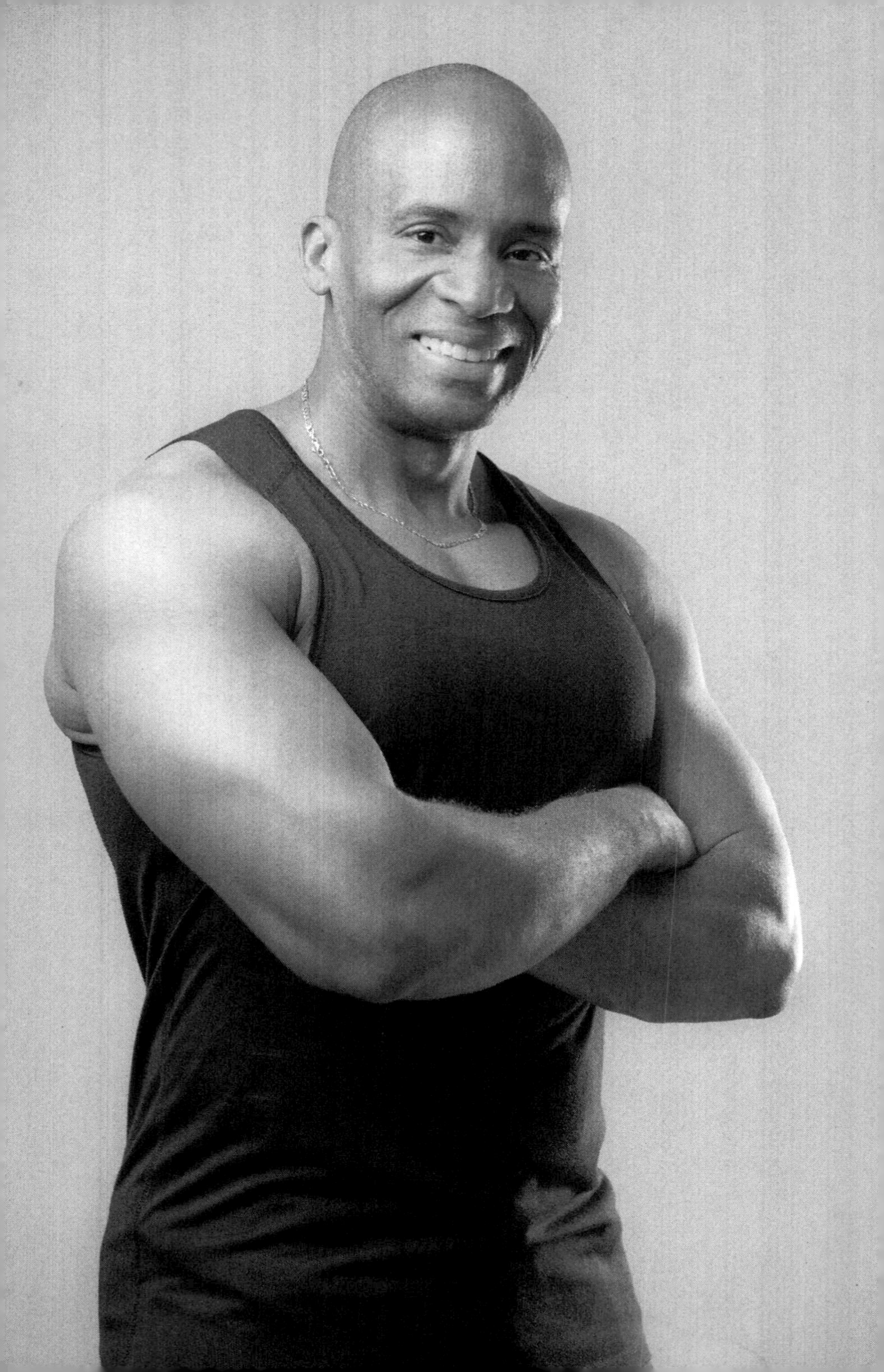

CHAPTER 1

Forbidden Fruit

"Rich, fatty foods are like destiny: they too, shape our ends."
- Author Unknown

I recently read a phenomenal book entitled "Faith & Fat Loss" by Ron Williams. It is a book that teaches you how to transform your life both physically and spiritually in 21 days by taking you through the history of how bad food choices affected the people living in Biblical times – beginning with Adam and Eve. I find myself captivated by the food choice made by Eve in the Garden of Eden and how that one choice has had such a major impact on humanity today! Eve was deceived; she was seduced and persuaded by Satan to eat the Forbidden Fruit. Eve made a bad choice. God had given Adam and Eve the liberty to occupy the entire garden for their pleasure with just one exception, and that was eating from the Tree of Knowledge. Their decision to eat from the tree reaped havoc on future generations.

Genesis 3:4-6
"You will not surely die," the serpent said to the woman, "for God knows that when you eat of it your eyes will be opened, and you will be like God, knowing good and evil." When the woman saw that the fruit of the

> ***tree was good for food and pleasing to the eye, and also desirable for gaining wisdom, she took some and ate it. She also gave some to her husband, who was with her, and he ate it.***

After reading the book, I realized that we are still paying the price for Eve's choice in the garden today and it prompted me to think about the struggles so many of us have with our food choices on a daily basis. In many ways, we are still paying the price for some of the food choices our ancestors made. However, in some instances, they were not to blame. Throughout history, slaves are known to have had a very limited and unhealthy diet. In fact, they were forced to eat the scraps and leftovers from their slave owners in order to survive. Because of this, slaves had to become very creative with the little they had to be able to feed their families and this resulted in what we know today as "soul food." Of course, we also know today that most soul food is high in cholesterol and saturated fats, two ingredients that are major contributors in many diet related health problems, including America's number one killer, heart disease. Many adults today suffer from high blood pressure because of eating habits they were taught as a child. Some of us have inherited cardiovascular related issues, hypertension, diabetes and high blood pressure because of hereditary food choices. We are no longer forced to make these food choices for our very survival, so what's our excuse for continuing to make them today?

The answer is, we are constantly bombarded by advertisements, books, programs, health experts, doctors, nutritionists and countless others, all telling us about the proper food choices we should be making to enhance our lives as well as advising us of the foods that are detrimental to our well being – such as chips, chocolate, pastries, soft drinks, and fast foods. Many fad diets and so called weight loss programs promise to make us feel better, satisfy our tastes, and reap long term benefits. But, have you been deceived? When Eve was deceived by Satan, she was not only motivated by his words but by the appearance of the fruit itself, it looked pleasing to her. How many times have your senses been stimulated by a tempting food commercial or a graphic, descriptive restaurant menu? Have you ever noticed that the food you order from the restaurant menu never looks the picture when it's on your plate? Why is that? ***DECEPTION!*** I sometimes ask my server why the meal doesn't look like the picture on the menu and they—just laugh.

We can't let the media control our senses or our appetite. We should use our own eyes to read food labels and see for ourselves which foods represent good food choices. This means learning to recognize the ingredients that are not good for us and to identify the foods that contain harmfully high amounts of unhealthy elements such as high fructose corn syrup and mono-sodium L-glutamate, better known as MSG. Somewhat incredibly, these harmful ingredients are in 95 percent of the processed foods we consume, making them almost impossible to avoid. However, the more knowledgeable we become about the foods we eat and the more we understand about individual ingredients, the closer we can get to eliminate this poison from our diets all together. One simple way to cut down the consumption of potentially harmful ingredients is to cut back on the consumption of highly processed foods. Another way is to completely avoid the consumption of all "fast foods," but for many of us, this is not as simple as it sounds. I know it may be hard, but remember this – fast food may lead you to a faster death!

Don't Be Deceived

Let me take a minute here to incorporate some practical ways to reverse the curse and to share some ideas that will help to put you on the right track to becoming a healthier you.

- Start reading labels on products and avoid foods and drinks that contain high fructose corn syrup and MSG when possible.
- Prepare more home cooked meals. At least you will know what's in it!
- Plan to eat smaller meals more often. This will help you to avoid making unhealthy choices "on the go."
- Never go food shopping on an empty stomach!
- Beware of fad diets and rapid weight loss programs. Use the FDA (Food and Drug Administration) Food Pyramid Chart as your food guideline.
- Drink at least 64 fluid ounces of water every day to avoid dehydration and prevent hunger. As a general guide, an average sized soft drink glass holds around 8 fluid ounces of water.
- Take a multi-vitamin daily to help your body get its proper nutrients.
- Eat more organic fruits and vegetables when possible.
- Educate yourself on what types of foods are good for you.
- Find an accountability partner to help you make good nutritional choices.
- And commit to exercising a minimum of three times a week!

Too Much or Too Little of a Good Thing?

Deception can lead to making bad food choices. Clever marketing campaigns and persuasive advertising can lead you into believing every word of the "message" they have been carefully crafted to send. The more high profile the product being promoted, the more convinced you become that everything the promoters say *must* be true. Have you ever been led into trying a product because a particular celebrity endorsed it? Have you ever gone on a diet because it was promoted as the diet used by one of your favorite celebrities—who happens to be in great shape? Chances are you have; and chances are things did not work out the way the marketing material promised. You were deceived. Just like Eve in the Garden of Eden, you were seduced and persuaded by the "promises" being made.

When it comes to eating a healthy diet, many women associate the word "diet" with deprivation. It's a mistaken belief that eating healthily means eating next to nothing or that all the foods you love to eat will become "forbidden fruit." This is simply not true. A healthy diet is a **balanced** diet, not a diet restricted to lettuce leaves or herbal tea. Your diet must be varied in order to obtain all of the nutrients your body needs so in many cases, getting the balance right can mean eating **more** of certain food types, not just eating less of everything. To be able to make good food choices, you must recognize that you do have a choice. Okay, you may not be at liberty to choose a chocolate filled donut but that's not your *only* choice; you can choose some strawberries or a banana smoothie instead. Or how about a piece of fruit bread, a rice cake, a bowl of cherries or—the list goes on? To be successful in changing your eating habits, you must change the way you think and keep your focus on what you ***can*** have, not what you ***can't.***

The problem with most fad diets is that they promise a "quick fix" and although it is possible to lose weight rapidly by following a restrictive diet plan, it's not a healthy way to lose weight and it's not a permanent way to keep the weight off. If you severely limit your daily intake of calories, your body effectively goes into starvation mode and it begins to do whatever it can to conserve energy. This means your body begins to use muscle as its energy source and the rate at which your body burns calories actually slows down. When you then inevitably return to more "normal," less restrictive eating habits, you will quickly regain any weight you lost. If your eating habits are unhealthy, you will gain even more. Radical fad diets simply don't work, not only because of the way your body physically responds but also because of the way you are most likely to respond psychologically. The more restrictive your diet is, the more you will begin to fixate on all of the things you *can't* have and your focus will become negative. It takes positive thoughts to generate positive actions and it takes positive actions to generate positive outcomes. To be effective *and* permanent, changes to your diet and lifestyle must be made gradually.

Pros and Cons of Popular Quick Fixes

Two of the most popular "quick fix" diets are the cabbage soup diet and detox diets. Here is a quick look at the pros and cons.

Cabbage Soup Diet

Pros: It's a diet plan that lasts only seven days and if you stick with the plan, weight loss is almost guaranteed. The food choices available represent healthy choices, especially if you have been eating a diet of high sugar and high fat foods. It's easy to follow and relatively inexpensive, and you don't get hungry because you can eat as much soup as you want.
Cons: The weight loss over the seven day period is mainly water loss. The caloric intake is low and the full range of nutrients needed by the body is

not provided which can lead to low energy levels, feelings of weakness or health issues such as headaches. It's also boring!

Detox Diets

Pros: Like the cabbage soup diet, the food choices available on most detox diets represent healthy food choices. The intake of fresh fruits, vegetables and water combined with the elimination of processed foods and toxins such as caffeine can lead to an improved overall sense of well-being as well as weight loss.

Cons: The extremely limited range of foods permitted on most detox diets fail to provide the body with a healthy balance of nutrients which can lead to low levels of energy, health issues such as light-headedness and poor concentration, and feelings of hunger leading to unhealthy food cravings.

The best fix is always a slow and steady fix with gradual changes being the only effective way to make *lasting* changes to your diet and lifestyle.

Most habits, eating habits included, are habits of a lifetime so it's unrealistic to expect to be able to stick with any plan that represents a radical change away from what you currently do. Scientific research has concluded that it takes a period of at least 21 days to change a habit, meaning that new habits can be formed as well as old habits dropped by remaining consistent with the change being made on a daily basis over a three week period. My 21 day program is designed to do just that by getting you into the *habit* of exercising and making healthy food choices without making unrealistic, dramatic changes that are unsustainable.

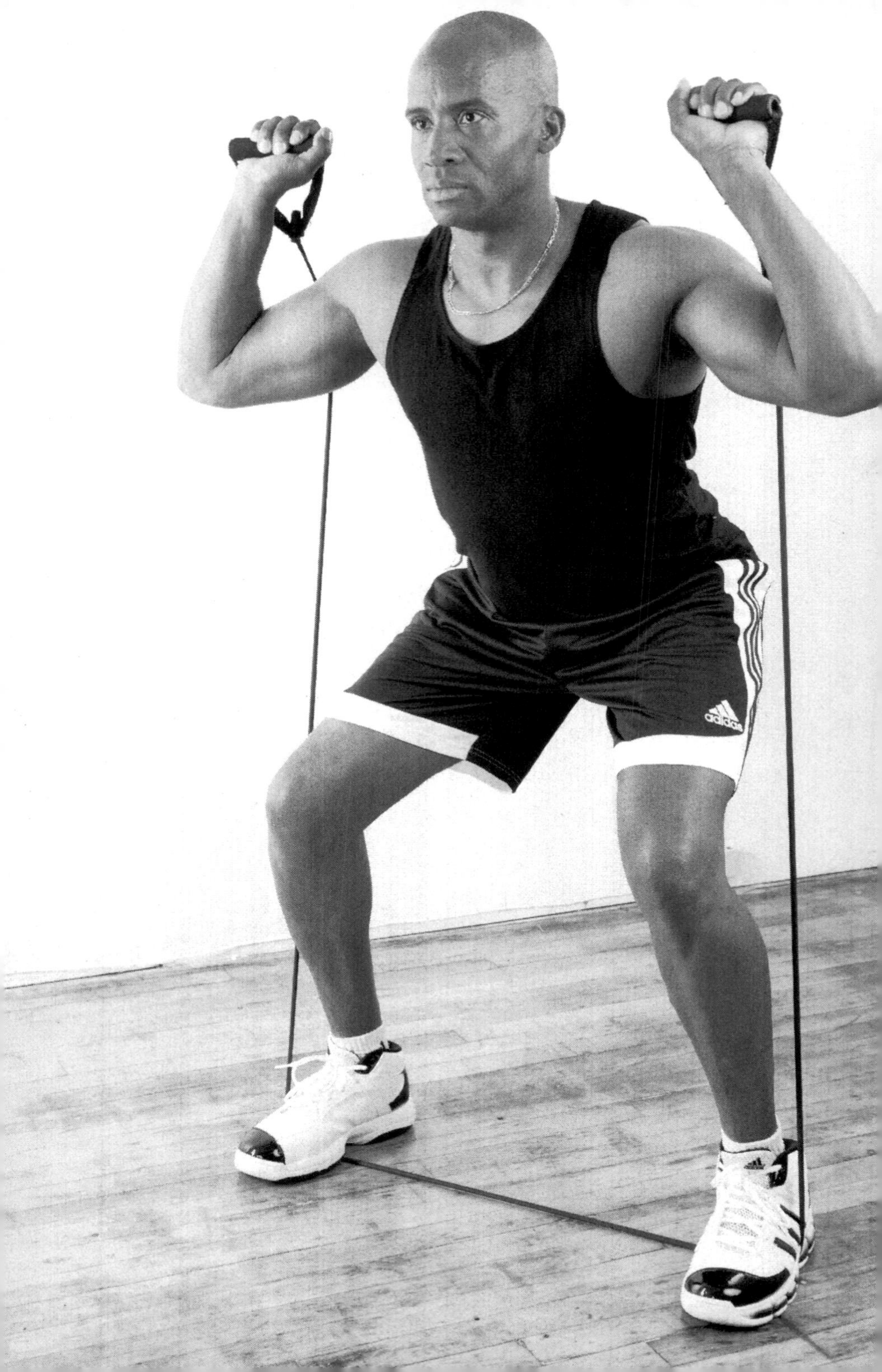
adidas

CHAPTER 2

From Hell to Good Health

"Gluttony is an emotional escape, a sign something is eating us."
- Peter De Vries

All things are possible through Christ! Now you may have different spiritual beliefs, but I just have to share with you what worked for me. No matter what you believe in, most people agree that there is someone much greater and more powerful than we are. This program will help you get in shape no matter where you are spiritually, but I feel compelled to tell you about my source of strength and to give credit where it's due. I can in no way take the credit for what God has delivered me from and what he has brought me through.

Being known in most circles as a Health and Fitness Expert, my story may shock you. About 20 years ago I lived a life of destruction: I was headed to an early grave and probably straight to Hell. I wasted three years of my life smoking crack cocaine and partying every weekend. I could drink most people under the table and most times that's where I ended up—UNDER THE TABLE!
Unfortunately, I secretly carried this stronghold and demon into my marriage and it was an ongoing struggle to defeat the demons within. Many times, just when it seemed that I had overcome this challenge,

something traumatic would happen in my life to trigger my return to a downward spiral of destructive behavior. It was so depressing to fall again and again without having someone to talk to who could identify with my situation. Secret sin is the worst kind because it puts you in a state of denial.

Satan was trying to destroy me!

John 10:10

"The thief cometh not, but for to steal, and to kill, and to destroy; I am come that they might have life, and they might have it more abundantly." Satan.

Throughout my personal training career, I have come to realize that most people have some type of issue that affects their well-being. Most addictive behaviors stem from unresolved issues from the past so the first step to living a healthy life is to discover and address the root of your problem. Exercise has some value, but good health starts from the inside out.

1Timothy 4:8

For bodily exercise profited little; but godliness is profitable unto all things, having promise of the life that now is, and of that which is to come.

So with that said, what is your vice? Whether it's drugs, alcohol, chocolate, caffeine or sweets, addiction involves a substance over which you feel you have no control. Over a period of time, whether it's narcotics or food, they are all substances that can negatively affect your health and ultimately may one day kill you. In some aspects, a food addiction can be worse than a drug addiction because you don't have to run to the liquor store or the drug dealer: You can just open up your refrigerator or your cupboards and get your fix there and then. Food is a legal drug and I believe that sugar is the number one leading legal drug in America. It's a drug that's readily available to all of us and you don't have to look far to find it because sugar, whether artificial or natural, can be found in just about everything. For some of us, going only a day or two without sugar can generate a dramatic change in mood, attitude and personality because we are essentially withdrawing from a drug. So the next time you find yourself judging someone who may be addicted to narcotics, take a look at the mirror and ask yourself – "do you have any legal addictions?" If an honest answer reveals that you do and you realize that you need to find an escape route, let me share with you the escape route from addiction that worked for me.

Before I was able to transform my life from Hell to good health, I had to have an encounter with the one and only transformer, Jesus the Christ. He brought me through my alcohol addiction, my drug addiction *and* my addiction with food!

> **2 Corinthians 5:17**
> ***Therefore, if any man be in Christ, he is a new creature; old things are passed away; behold, all things become new.***

Many fitness programs promise their clients transformation without the transformer – and they inevitably always end with disappointing results. God has now brought me to a place where I feel bad if I eat a chicken box or drink a can of soda and for me that is true transformation; and it's a transformational power that only God can provide. I believe that if you're struggling with your diet or weight, you would do well to consider turning it over to the one who can fix it. God has used exercise as a tool to keep many people on track and focused. I know he has used it for me and I know it has worked. Exercise will equip you with self-control and purpose, and it is also a great way to relieve stress.

It has worked for me!
Weight and cardiovascular training have become my ultimate high—
IT IS THE BEST FREE HIGH I HAVE EVER KNOWN!
I feel great now when I am on a regular workout program and so will you.

Some diet and fitness programs will give you temporary results, however, when we include God into our program, change is permanent. You've tried everything else, what do you have to lose?

God wants us to be in good health, he says it in his word.

> **3 John 1:2**
> ***Beloved, I wish above all things that you may prosper and be in health, even as your soul prospers.***

Overcoming a Stronghold

The first step towards overcoming a stronghold is simply to *take that first step.* Listed below are some tips that will help you to take that all important step and continue to support you on your journey to a healthier you.

- Ask God to intervene in your situation.
- Find an accountability partner.

- Avoid stress in your life as much as possible.
- Surround yourself with people who encourage and motivate you.
- Set monthly goals that will challenge you.
- Find a scripture and stand on the word of God for your breakthrough.
- Get involved in a physical activity to keep you fit and occupied.
- Avoid people in your life that are bad influences until you become stronger.
- Prepare healthy meals ahead of time and drink plenty of water.
- Recognize your weaknesses and avoid distractions.

Good health is not a trip, it's a lifelong journey.

Have you already attempted to work out and then fallen short just before you reached your goal? That's no reason to stop your efforts to get fit or give up on your goals. No overnight program will shed away extra pounds and keep them off. Staying steady and consistent is the only way to accomplish your mission so the key to success is to make improving your health and fitness a fun and enjoyable process. Find a deeper source of motivation; a deeper reason to stick with it that goes beyond outward benefits, and this will carry you through the tough times. Surround yourself with positive people who will give you the encouragement you need when you need it most and avoid negativity at *all* cost!

Getting There

You can't get to where you're going if you don't know where you're coming from – and until you know exactly where it is you're going to, it's impossible to know whether you have arrived! Confused? Let me explain: My own journey took me from Hell to good health but it was a journey that could not begin until I recognized I was not where I wanted *to* be. I was in the wrong place and I realized I needed to be someplace else, but where? I had to figure out where the right place for me was; I had to know what this place called "good health" was going to look like for me in my life before I could take steps to get there. Just like a car journey, you have to know exactly where you are and exactly where you want to be in order to find the best route between the two points.

Three Things You Can Do Right Now to Get Started

1. JOT DOWN YOUR PLAN

Set realistic goals and identify a person to keep you on track. Focus on where you want to be and not where you are. Use pictures and positive affirmations to help you.

Motivational goals and inspirational people:

____
____
____
____
____
____
____
____
____
____

2. EAT WITH WISDOM

Gradually change your eating habits. Baby steps are better than no steps at all. Add fruits and vegetables to your nutritional plan, this will help you feel better within a few weeks. You are what you eat and drink, so drink plenty of water each day. This will curve your appetite and help your metabolism work more effectively.

Fruits and vegetables I like or would like to try:

____

____

____

____

____

____

____

____

____

____

3. GET ACTIVE

Changing your eating habits and making positive life changes are good, but without physical activity you are still imbalanced. When you are totally fit in Mind, Body and Spirit, nothing can stand in your way!

Activities I like or would like to try:

____

____

____

____

____

____

____

____

Staying There

America is rebounding from a recession and to make matters worse we are right smack in the middle of a serious obesity epidemic. Although finances are important, money cannot replace good health. God's favor will go further than money ever will. The media continues to bombard us with advertisements promoting weight loss, encouraging us to buy into the latest products and programs, yet our obesity rate is steadily increasing; why is that?

The older I get, the more I realize that people have so much in common. With society moving at such a fast pace, we tend to get distracted and bored easily. Whether it's going from church to church, job to job or relationship to relationship, we've been wired to expect instant gratification. If we don't get it, we eagerly explore other options. If we continue down this path, we will never reach our goals and have true peace. Consistency is one of the essential building blocks to success. If your desire is to have permanent good health, it's going take a consistent plan to achieve that; it's only by doing the right things consistently over a period of time that you can expect to reap the results you desire. You reap what you sow.

So how do we stay motivated after the initial excitement of beginning an exercise program has worn off? The answer is to make exercise fun. It stands to reason that the more you enjoy an activity, the more likely you are to keep doing it. By sticking with it and being consistent, you will soon begin to notice improvements and those improvements, along with the fact that it's fun, provide you with all the motivation you need to keep going. The 21 day plan I share with you in this book begins with baby steps which start you on your way to creating new habits. Once you create good habits, in terms of both eating and workout habits, fitness becomes a way of life and a routine. It's having a **routine** of good habits that helps us to conquer future health challenges.

Walk it Off

A pedometer walking program is a good way to begin your journey from where you are now to where you want to be and it compliments the "I'm Too Cute to Sweat" routine. Walking is not as intensive as jogging or cycling, therefore it is necessary to exercise for a longer period of time in order to burn the same number of calories you might during a shorter but more intense exercise session. Of course, if you're too cute to sweat, walking is a great "low sweat" alternative to running, but believe me when I say that power walking is definitely a fat burner. During 30 minutes of walking, you would normally take approximately 4,000 steps, burning about 200 calories. If losing a few pounds is your goal, then your walk would need to be quite intensive, as only then will your heart rate stay at the optimum level to aid fat burning. However, at any intensity, the further you walk the more calories you will burn. Fitting a long walk into your busy schedule may not seem like an instantly manageable task but there are always alternative ways to fit exercise into your life. For example, a walk of one and a half hours per day may not be a practical option but how about three half hour walks spread throughout the day? Where there is a will, there is *always* a way.

A pedometer is rather inexpensive, prices vary depending on the number of functions and overall quality, but a basic model is all you need to get started. It's a simple device that can be worn comfortably around your wrist, although it's more accurate if it's placed around your waist just above your hips where it's more likely to recognize every step you take. All in all, a pedometer is an accessible, easy and effective way to add interest and meaning to a walking program.

First, you will need to find out how many steps it takes you to walk to work, to the supermarket, to the park with the kids or anywhere you normally go on foot. Start a log where you can record the total number of steps taken each day, as well as the distance, time and the routes you take. By doing so for at least a week, you will be able to analyze the distance and the time you currently walk. You now have all the information you need to begin making beneficial adjustments—you know where you're coming from. The adjustments you make will depend on where it is you now want to go. If it's your goal to walk 10,000 or 12,000 steps each day, you can now look at ways of adjusting your current routine to begin building up from where you are to where you want to be. This might mean taking a slightly longer route to work or walking an extra circuit or two around the pond in the park when you're out for a walk with your baby in the buggy. It might take a little imagination to begin with but you will soon notice yourself actively looking for ways to increase your daily number of steps so that your pedometer can record your efforts. Choose any opportunity to walk more on a daily basis. Take the stairs instead of the elevator, park your car at the furthest point in the parking lot or park in the lot that's a block away from the building you're going to and walk back. Remember to keep your log records up-to-date. Your records will not only help you to recognize the most beneficial routes, keeping track of the improvements you are making will also give your motivation a real boost and encourage further activity. Walking is one of the safest ways to improve your health, to get fit and to *stay* fit and healthy, no matter what your size or fitness level.

All of us, whether we are big or small, are at risk from cardiovascular disease; this problem is universal. Good health can only be improved by moderate exercise and making wise nutritional choices. That's a fact! A study published in the ***Journal of the American Medical Association*** concluded that low-fat diets DO NOT, despite all of the hype, reduce a woman's risk of cancer or heart disease, **only regular exercise will do that.**

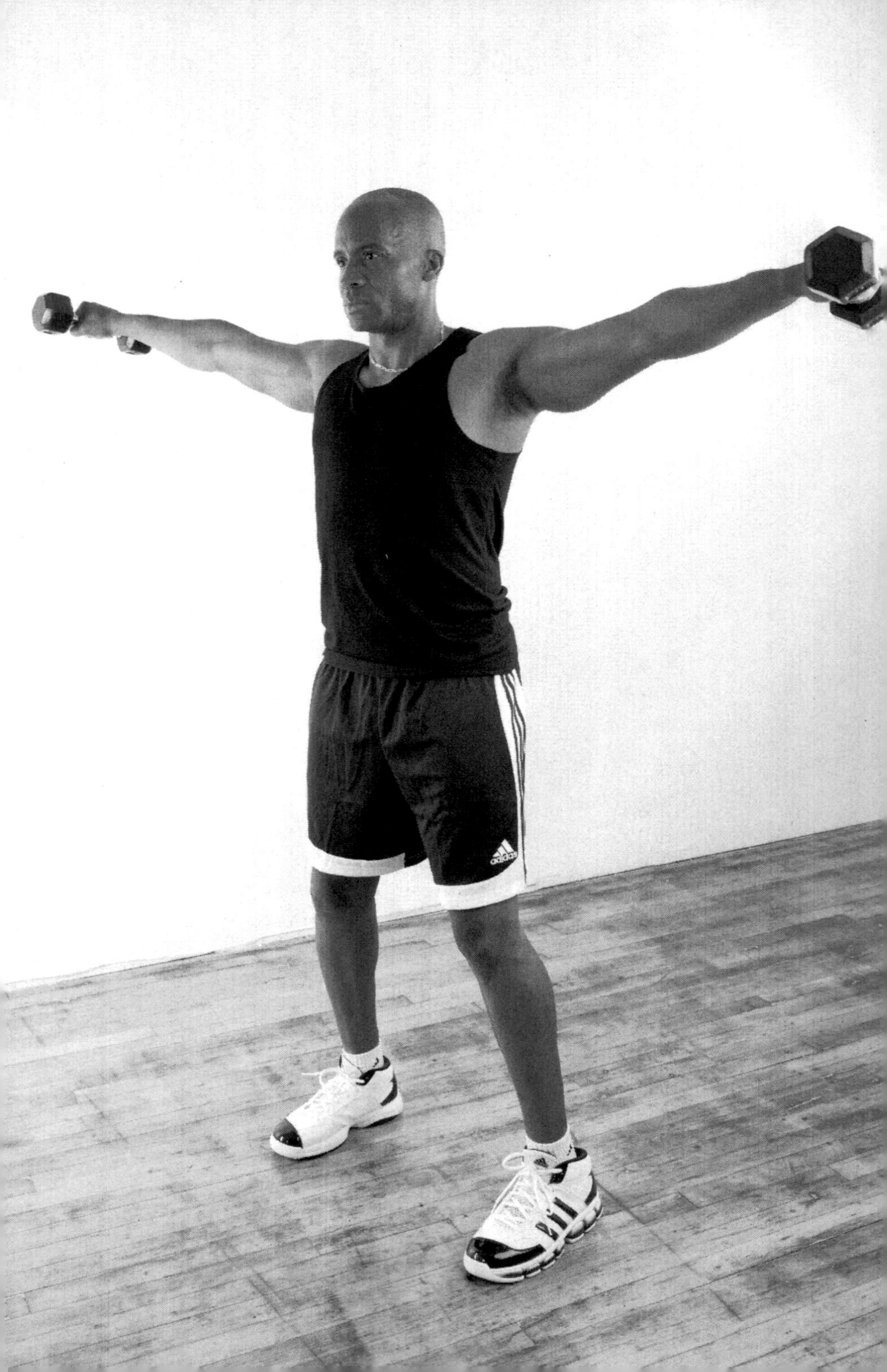

Chapter 3

Your Health is Your Wealth

"The greatest wealth is health."
- Virgil

Did you know that a study once revealed thin people earn more money than obese people? That is why I believe that your health is your wealth; not only for that reason, but also because Americans spend large quantities of time away from work due to sickness and health related issues. Many of these sick days are taken without pay, simply because many sick banks have been depleted.

Did you know that being overweight is not equivalent to being unfit? In fact, being underweight actually kills over 30,000 Americans a year. So why do Americans continue to buy into the idea that thinner is better? Even though diets prove to be ineffective 95 percent of the time, we spend 40 billion dollars annually on diet products. Studies also show that 7 million women suffer from eating disorders; 35 percent of those who diet go on to yo-yo dieting, which is more unhealthy than being overweight, and 25 percent of those who diet tend to develop some type of severe eating disorder.

Are You Living a Healthy Lifestyle?

Answer the following 10 questions—be totally honest with yourself!

1. Do you spend more than four hours a day watching television?
2. Do you eat at fast-food restaurants at least five times a week?
3. Do you find yourself tired even after a full night of sleep?
4. Do you have a busy or stressful life?
5. Do you experience shortness of breath when you climb more than one flight of stairs?
6. Do you make excuses or procrastinate when it comes to exercise?
7. Do you plan your meals in advance or do you eat whatever, whenever?
8. Do you eat less than four meals a day?
9. Have you noticed a decline in your energy level over the years?
10. Have you noticed that you are not as flexible as you used to be?

If you have answered *"yes"* to any of these questions, you may want to address some of these areas in your life. Take small steps each day to improve each of them and it would help to have an accountability partner to keep you on track. The first step to making changes in your life is admitting that you need help. Don't be afraid to talk with a Certified Fitness Trainer and/or a Nutritionist to get you started.

The economy is tight, but you can still make it happen. The time is now and this is the perfect opportunity to get back to the fundamentals of life by enjoying family and friends. Hang in there – your breakthrough is coming! If you are considering eliminating some luxuries, don't let fitness be one of them. Make taking care of your health a top priority. In fact, there are many ways to use these tough times to your advantage.

A healthy lifestyle is essential because it helps relieve stress and release endorphins to keep us emotionally stable and happy. The last thing we need right now, or at any time, is to lie around and let our surroundings consume us. I always say, it's hard for the devil to hit a moving target and that is why I believe it is so important to get involved with activities that make you feel good and boost your self-esteem.

Staying healthy and being active does not have to be an expensive journey. You can join a walking club or partake in a group fitness class in your community, a free and easy way to lose weight and/or maintain your well-being. Your local recreation center or YMCA is a great place to find fun and affordable activities year round, and cycling is another great way to enjoy the outdoors and keep fit - it's also cheap on gas! From a nutritional stand point, most people eat better during summer. It is the perfect season to take some time off from the kitchen and grill your meats and vegetables. This too will help you look and feel healthier. Before leaving the house, make sure you carry some water and healthy snacks with you. This will help cut down on drinking fatty beverages and making bad food choices, as well as cutting down on unnecessary expenses. Getting into the habit of eating smaller proportioned meals throughout the day will boost your metabolism and prevent you from impulse eating or impulse buying which usually results in unhealthy food choices.

Affordable Ways to Stay Healthy

Here are a few more ways to stay healthy without blowing the budget.

- Get involved with a walking or running group at work, church, or in your community.

- Find an enjoyable hobby and stick with it. (Walking, photography, gardening, etc.)
- Get a fitness trainer and split the cost with some friends.
- Prepare your food at home and avoid eating fast foods.
- Drink plenty of water throughout the day and avoid carbonated beverages.
- Give back to the community by donating your time to a youth group.
- Get some fitness DVDs and work out at home.
- Grill your meals and vegetables instead of cooking them on the traditional stove.
- Take time to do something for YOU!
- Spend some quite time to rest, relax, and meditate!

If you are new to exercise and your goal is to shed some excess fat, it's not a good plan to focus too much on what your scales are telling you. Your scales can help you track pounds lost, but you don't know if those pounds are actually fat or muscle. A better way to evaluate your progress is by how your clothes fit or by a sudden flow of compliments! Muscle weighs more than fat and you could be gaining muscle while also losing fat, so don't become obsessed with the number on the scale; the scale is not a true gauge. Let the way you feel be your motivation. Remember, you need to look after your health because your health is your wealth!

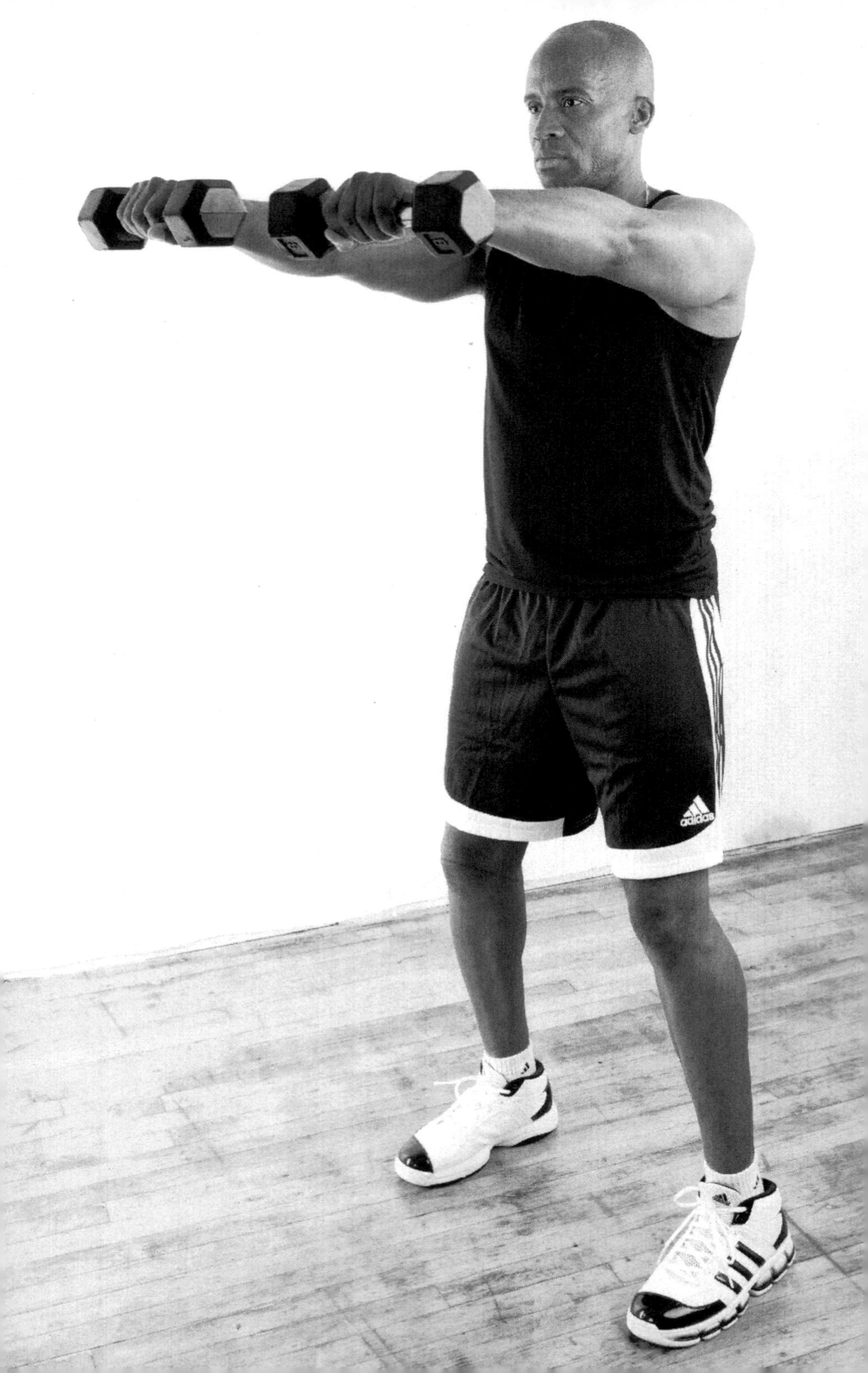
adidas

Chapter 4

Nutrition to Control Your Weight

"Never eat more than you can lift."
- Miss Piggy

Nutritionists often talk about the foods you shouldn't eat in order to promote a healthy lifestyle but in this chapter, we're going to discuss what you *should* eat and how to combine the proper micro-nutrients to help aid fat loss. First of all, micro-nutrients are your proteins, carbohydrates, and essential fatty acids. When you eat these nutrients in the right combination, they will help you burn fat more rapidly. About 90 percent of our population at some point in time will have some concerns about their weight, especially their "gut" or that "spare tire" of fat that develops around the mid-section. Your metabolism is critical in terms of weight loss as it has a major role to play in how you shed the extra pounds, so it's important to understand a little more about it.

Your metabolism is like the motor of your body. It is the rate at which your body burns calories when at rest. Typically, we use 60-70 percent of our calories at our resting metabolic rate and we can burn more when we participate in physical activities. However, it isn't just extra activity that affects our metabolism; the amount of muscle tissue we have plays a major part on where the bulk of our calories are burned. Unfortunately, if you are not participating in a training program that utilizes weights, you will not maintain your lean muscle mass. The average person will lose approximately 1 ½ pounds of lean muscle every year, usually beginning around the age of 30. This means the more lean muscle mass you develop and maintain, the better your metabolism will function. In addition, weight training is essential for keeping the weight off once you reach your desired weight. Research has shown that people who lose weight through a combination of weight lifting, cardiovascular training and good nutrition are better able to keep off unwanted fat than those who only use fad diets.

The start of any successful exercise program is laying the proper nutritional foundation. Trying to start a regiment without the right balance of carbohydrates, proteins, fats, vitamins and minerals can be harmful to the body in the long term. These elements provide fuel for the body which not only fuels your workouts; it also helps your body maximize its potential during workout recovery.

Carbohydrates

Let's start with carbohydrates, often abbreviated to carbs. These provide the body with energy and they can be divided into two groups:

1. **Simple carbs** – sugary foods are included in this group and simple carbs are found in fruits and candy.
2. **Complex carbs** – starchy foods are included in this group and complex carbs are found in foods such as pasta and rice.

Although carbs are good for the body, too many can be a problem because they breakdown into sugar which then produces unwanted fat. One way to prevent this is to never eat a carbohydrate alone. Always eat your carbs with proteins and essential fatty acids as part of a balanced meal. It's actually best to eat carbohydrates before a training session for energy and afterwards to replenish but as a general rule, you should aim to get around 60 percent of your daily caloric intake from carbs.

Protein

Protein is the building block for muscle, providing the body with the necessary nutrients to help it repair itself after a vigorous workout. Good sources of proteins include meats, fish, and nuts. You should aim to get about 15 percent of your daily calories from proteins, ideally by eating just a small amount at every meal.

Fats

Fats normally get a bad rap because most people feel they are unhealthy to eat. However, not all fats are "bad" and they are actually a great source of energy, also providing a protective layer around the organs. Saturated fats are the unhealthy fats, found in foods such as dairy products and red meats. They are high in cholesterol which can clog your arteries, leading to high blood pressure and an increased risk of developing heart disease. On the other hand, mono-unsaturated and polyunsaturated fats, such as those found in oily fish, nuts and wheat germ oil are much healthier for you.

Vitamins and Minerals

Vitamins and minerals are essential for good health and proper growth. By eating a varied and balanced diet, you will help provide your body with the right mix but in addition, a regular supplement of vitamins can help boost your intake of essential nutrients where food falls short.

Be Prepared

The key is to always plan ahead. If you can prepare your meals at least two days in advance or identify healthy places to eat out in advance, you increase your chances of fueling your body properly. When you eat small meals on a regular basis, you avoid getting hungry and this will prevent you from making bad choices when hunger strikes, leading you back into the need for instant gratification. To realize the full benefits of living a healthier, more energized life, a good plan should consist of 60 percent nutrition, 30 percent fitness, and 10 percent rest. By following my 21 day program, you will have a well-balanced plan. Remember, it is important to absorb the correct combination of nutrients to lose weight, ***not*** starve yourself and deprive your body of what it needs.

Balanced Nutrition

The FDA Food Pyramid Chart is a great way to educate yourself into getting a healthy balance in your daily diet.

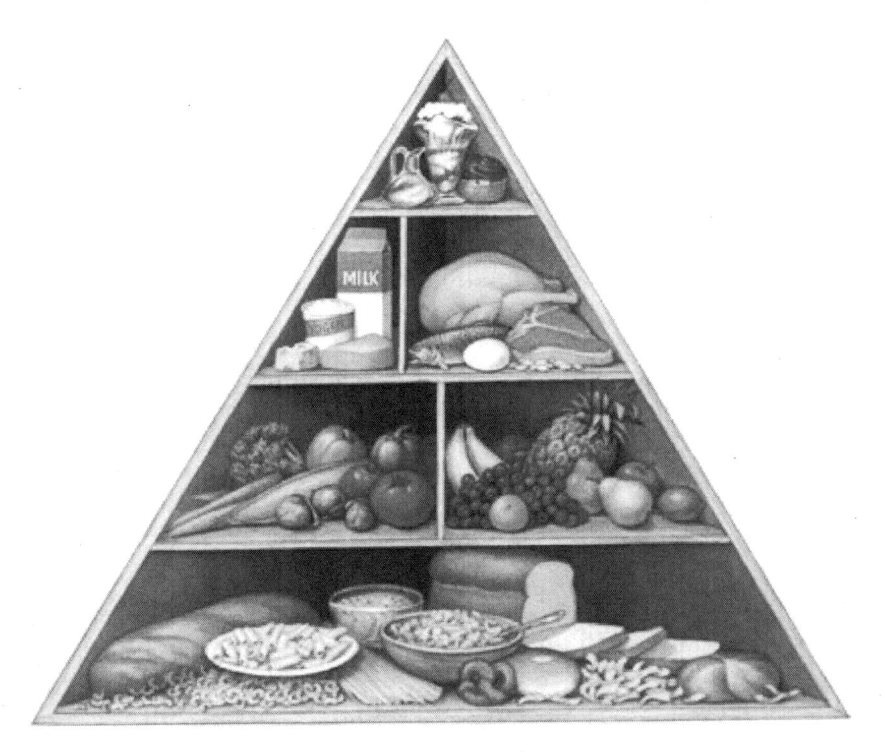

Food Pyramid

Tip the Balance

Listed below are some U.S. Department of Agriculture tips to help you tip the balance of your daily diet in a healthy direction:

- Avoid oversized portions.
- Enjoy your food but eat less.
- Make half your plate fruits and vegetables.
- Make at least half your grains whole grains.
- Switch to fat-free or low-fat milk.
- Choose foods with lower sodium content where possible.
- Drink water instead of sugary drinks.

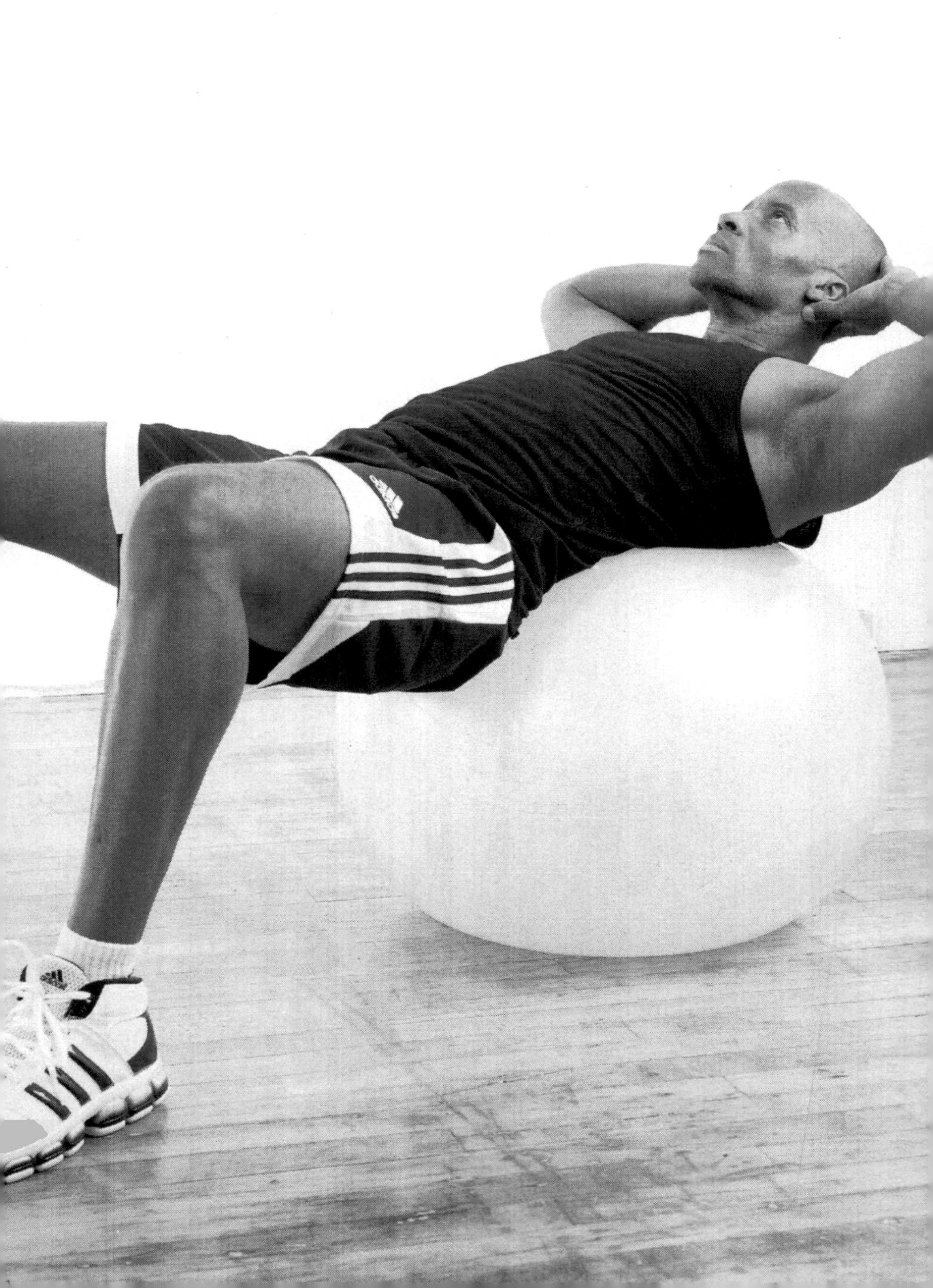

Chapter 5

Exercise Junkie

"My idea of exercise is a good brisk sit."
- Phyllis Diller

You may not consider yourself to be at this point yet or even imagine you ever will be, but believe it or not, once you start working out, you may become a fitness addict. Exercise addiction is rare, but it does exist. Some physiologists feel that a person can become addicted to exercise in much the same way that a person can become addicted to morphine. Vigorous exercise activities, such as intense power lifting or running, cause an increase in your endorphin levels. The word "endorphin" is a combination of two words; endogenous, meaning made in your body, and morphine. These two chemicals act on the same receptors in your body as narcotics, which is why some individuals feel "pumped up" after a really good workout. This endorphin "rush" is commonly known as a "runner's high" and it is one of the ways people can escape stress and clear their minds of life's daily pressures. A good workout can supply the same satisfaction for some as chocolate, nicotine or alcohol provides for others, explaining why someone can easily become addicted to exercise.

Intense exercise benefits us physically and psychologically. Another reason exercise may become addictive is that during intense exercise, endorphin levels are high and when endorphin levels become really high, it helps to block out physical and mental discomfort. This means our bodies produce more endorphins whenever we exert ourselves and the higher the levels, the more our bodies can tolerate pain.

Being an Exercise Junkie is great—but there is a negative side; compulsive exercise can consume all areas of a person's life.

People with this problem may find it impossible to stop training and they are often highly competitive. Even though they become fatigued or injured, they constantly strive to increase the intensity and length of their workouts. Another sign that a person may be flirting with a fitness addiction is that they begin to push everything else aside – family, friends, and other activities.

Are You a Compulsive Exerciser?

Listed below are 10 questions that will help you to identify whether you, or someone you know, may already be a compulsive exerciser – or be in danger of becoming one.

1. If you are not in the gym, do you daydream about exercise?
2. Do you push yourself to work out even though you have an injury?
3. Do you work out seven days a week?
4. Do you look forward to being sore the day after your workout?
5. Do you plan all other activities around your workout schedule?
6. Does most of your wardrobe consist of workout attire and sneakers?
7. Have your family and friends called you a workout fanatic?
8. Do you get depressed if you miss a day or two from the gym?
9. When you wake in the morning, is fitness the first thing you think

about?
10. Do you find yourself constantly looking in the mirror?

If you answered "*yes*" to one or more of the above questions, I applaud you for taking the necessary steps to improving your health. But, it's important to look at the "big picture" and to create a good balance in your life. Remember, allowing your body adequate rest and recovery time is a major component of being healthy and too much of a good thing *can* become a bad thing. I personally use fitness to help me control other bad habits in my life and it may become the same for you. If that's the case, go on and continue but just be aware that too much of anything, even exercise, is not good for you!

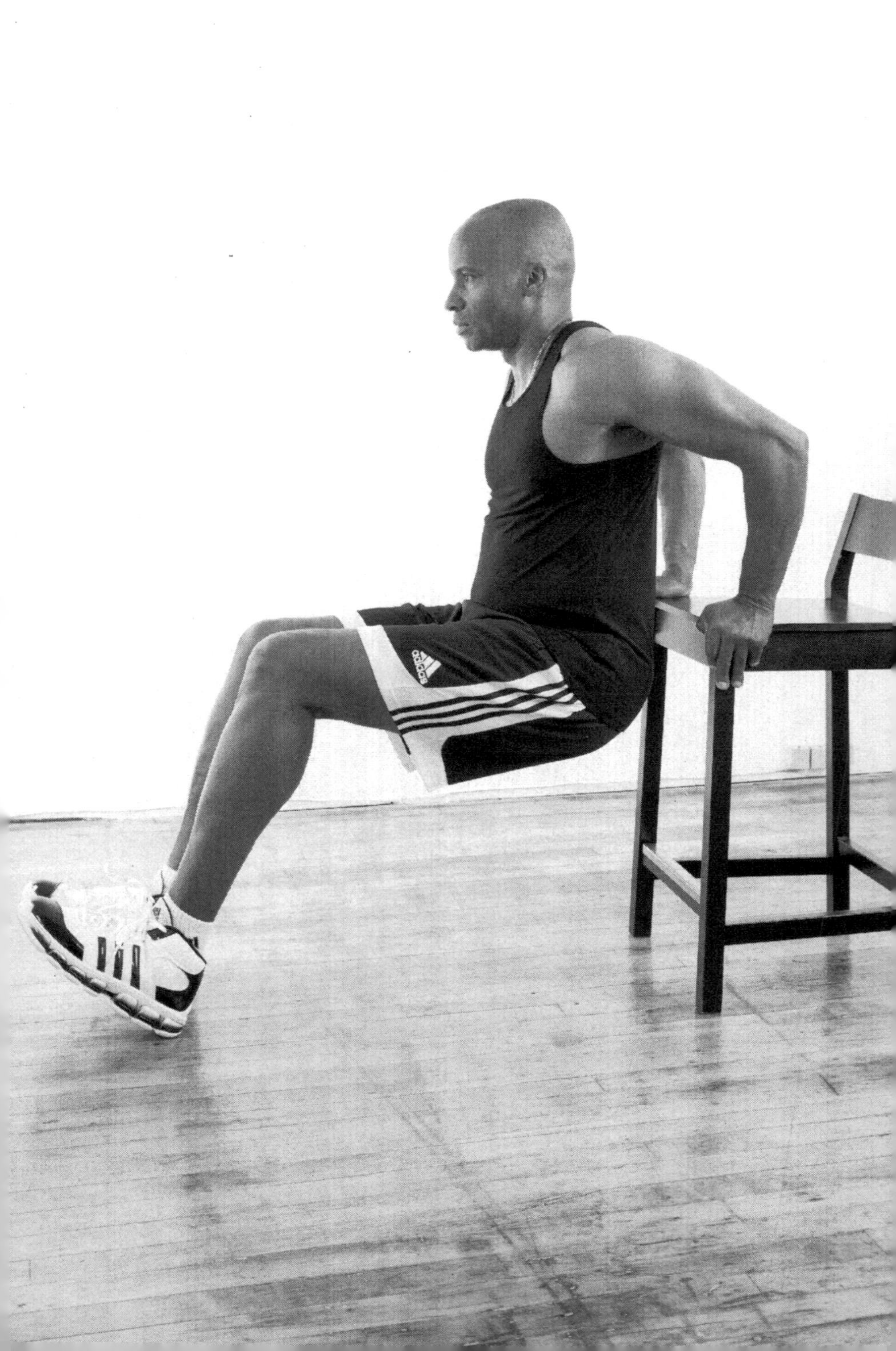
adidas

Chapter 6

It Hurts So Good

"Aerobics: a series of strenuous exercises which help convert fats, sugars and starches into aches, pains and cramps."

- Author Unknown

You may shy away from exercise because of the expected pain that follows a vigorous workout. Exercising is not a painless journey. We all have heard the cliché, "No Pain No Gain," and this not only holds true in the fitness arena, but in all areas of life whether it's spiritual, educational or physical, growth can be quite painful. The way forward is to accept that pain is unavoidable and to look for ways to make the growth process manageable and enjoyable. This is something I can help you with. The program you are about to embark upon consists of things that you are most likely doing in your daily life already. You will experience some slight discomfort in the beginning of this process, pain is unavoidable, and many of my clients ask me why exercise hurts and why a workout makes them sore. This is the reason why:

Muscle Soreness

The type of muscle soreness experienced after exercise is known as delayed onset muscle soreness (DOMS) and it normally occurs anywhere from 12 to 48 hours after the muscles in question have been exercised.

It is most commonly experienced by newcomers to exercise but it can affect anyone embarking on a new exercise program or making dramatic changes in their existing program by increasing the intensity or adding new activities. The soreness is generally at its worst within the first two days following the activity and gradually subsides over the next few days. DOMS is thought to be a result of microscopic tearing of the muscle fibers but scientific research has yet to discover the exact cause in all cases. It's known that the amount of tearing and therefore the degree of soreness you experience depends on how intensely you exercise, the duration of your exercise session and the type of exercises you do. Any new or unfamiliar movements can lead to muscle soreness, but eccentric movement□where the muscles work while lengthening instead of shortening□has been proven to cause the greatest degree of soreness. The good news is that muscles adapt to new stresses being placed upon them and muscle soreness is no longer experienced when the exercises you perform become familiar. This highlights the importance of staying consistent in your workout program and making gradual, progressive changes as your body adapts.

So you may ask, is there any way to prevent muscle soreness? Nothing is proven effective, but some studies have found the following advice helpful. The only way to discover if any of it is effective for you is to try a few things out and see what happens. Of course, avoiding workouts all together would be one guaranteed way to eliminate soreness but this is not an option for you! Any one of the suggested methods below may help to reduce or relieve muscle soreness and you may find combining these methods will help multiply the overall effect, leading to a faster return to comfort and a quicker recovery time.

Methods of Relieving Muscle Soreness

Here are some ways to eliminate or reduce the pain of muscle soreness:

- **Ibuprofen**

Ibuprofen taken before a workout can significantly reduce post workout soreness in some people, even more effectively than the same medication taken post workout. Since Ibuprofen is an anti-inflammatory drug, it may help to reduce the swelling and inflammation that causes the pain.

- **Massage**

Massage has also been shown to reduce soreness from a workout, and speed recovery time. The massaging action can help to increase the blood flow, remove the waste products in the muscle and reduce the swelling. It can also stimulate the release of pain-relieving hormones and aid in the breakup of scar tissue in the muscle.

- **Light Exercise**

Active recovery in the form of lightly exercising the affected muscles or exercising a different, unaffected group of muscles can lead to an increase in blood flow and reduction in overall inflammation. Light exercise can also provide a beneficial light stretching effect.

- **Stretching**

Stretching the affected area for 12 to 15 minutes after a light warm up of cardiovascular work can also reduce soreness.

- **Progressive Training**

When you begin the "I'm Too Cute to Sweat 21 Day Workout" or any new weight lifting routine, use light weights and high reps (10-15) initially before gradually increasing the amount you lift over several weeks as your body begins to adapt.

- **Introduce New Activities Gradually**

Avoid making sudden changes in your exercise routine or making major changes in the type of exercise you do.

- **Increase Your Workload Gradually**

Avoid making sudden changes or major increases in your workouts in terms of duration or intensity. This means increasing the amount of time you exercise for or the amount of weight you use in your workouts gradually.

- **Low-impact Exercise**

Active recovery in the form of low-impact exercise the day after a more intensive workout has been proven to help relieve some muscle soreness. Examples of low-impact activities are walking, stationary biking and low level aerobics classes.

I realize that pain is not fun, and going through the process is challenging. Over time, muscle soreness will diminish, but it will never totally go away. Keep your focus on the many benefits of exercise and all the positive things that regular exercise will bring into your life.

Remember—No Pain, No Gain!

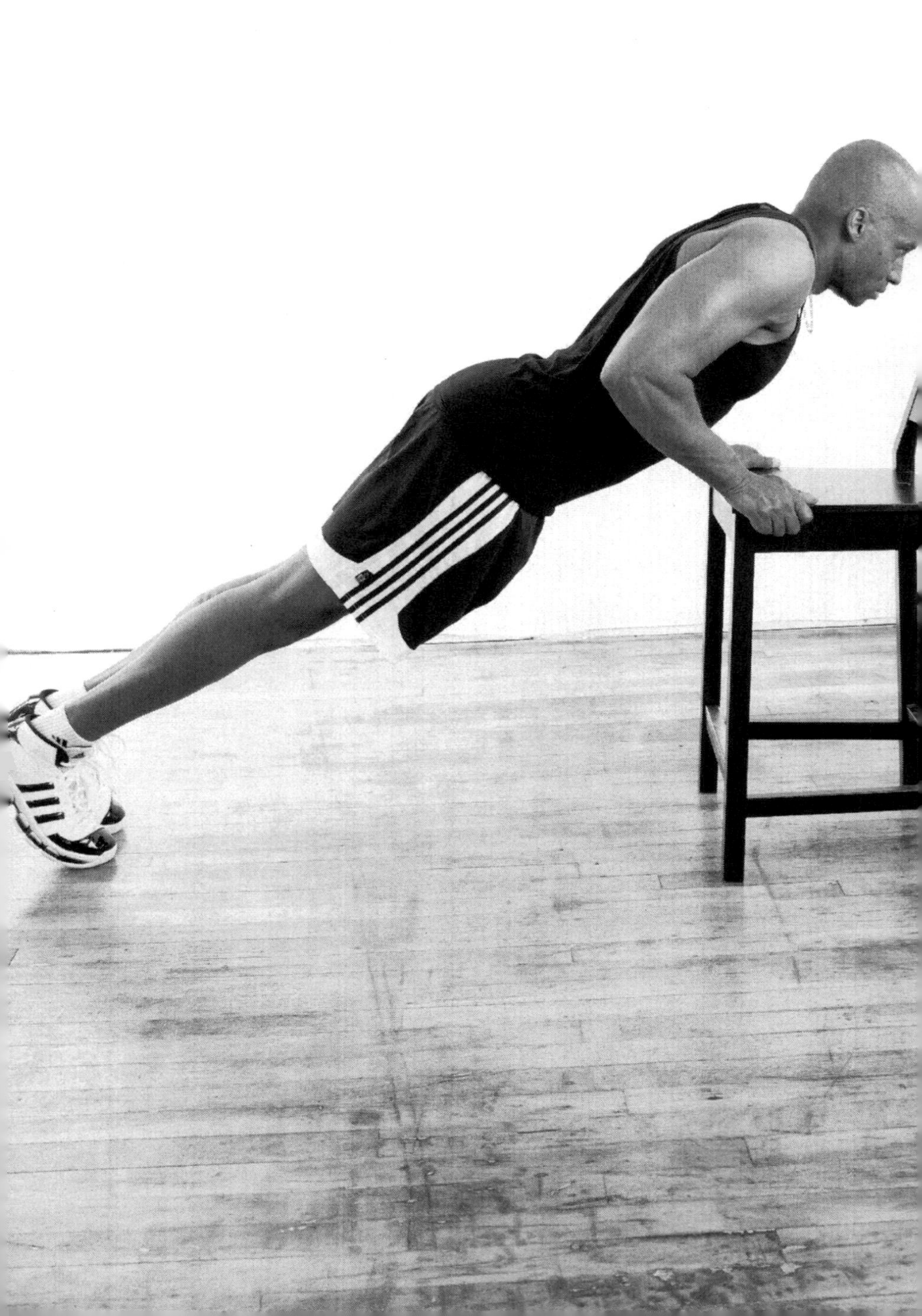

Chapter 7

The Size of a Sista

"A man's health can be judged by which he takes two at a time - pills or stairs."
- Joan Welsh

In the American culture, women come in all shapes, sizes and nationalities. Depending on your genetics – your body will vary in many ways. None of us are prisoners to our genetics, but there are some characteristics we can't change. We must agree that in some cases, African American and Hispanic women are genetically predisposed to having a shapely figure while other ethnic groups tend to have a "naturally" leaner physique. And that's okay!

Can we base good health on size alone?
Of course not!
Hollywood has given a false and unrealistic image of how the average woman should look.

While standing in the grocery line, we have all seen those American beauties who weigh no more than 100 pounds posing on the cover of the latest health and fitness magazine. Is that really healthy? No matter what your size or shape, your focus should always be on your health first and foremost and not on how much you weigh. Be honest with yourself and consider whether you currently put more effort into developing your outer appearance than you do building your self- image? The next question to ask is: What's more important – spirit or body? I believe we all know the answer to that question.

Let's take a brief inventory. On an annual basis, how much do you spend on cosmetics, nails, hair and entertainment? Now, how much do you spend on things that will help you grow? We have been blessed with a body that no other machine can match and it's our responsibility to take care of this gift. We must invest in taking care of ourselves and not destroy or abuse our bodies.

Poor nutrition and lack of exercise are the leading causes of obesity among women. What you put into your body may be your biggest stronghold. In our culture, we are raised on fried foods that are high in cholesterol and MSG and while those high fat foods may help you look curvier and bodacious for a little while, they will eventually lead to health problems and excess weight. Many times, it can seem that your body shape changes as soon as you hit 30 but these are not overnight changes, they are your past eating habits catching up with you. Even those size 8s can turn into double digits in a blink of an eye and you cannot continue to blame your weight on child birth when your youngest child is now in his/her freshman year of college. Having an hour glass shape is easily obtainable at any stage in your life with good nutrition, exercise and a healthy lifestyle.

I believe that because you are reading this book, this is *your* time to be fit.

Together we will achieve whatever your goals are. You will not only look good on the outside, you will also feel amazing on the inside. When you make wise choices to enhance your health, your true beauty will manifest on the outside. As you begin your journey through my 21 day program, I will be with you every step of the way.

Steps to Improving Your Health

Listed below are 10 small steps you can take to begin making BIG improvements in your health:

1. Love yourself for who you are.
2. Recognize the changes you need to make to improve your life and then strive to make them.
3. Look forward; don't let past fitness failure control your future.
4. Eat to feed your body and not your appetite.
5. Find an activity that you *enjoy* while also helping to burn calories.
6. Surround yourself with positive people.
7. Remain positive; do not give in to negative thoughts!
8. Find time to meditate and evaluate your life regularly.
9. Accept that it's not possible to please everyone—it's impossible to please God and man—don't be a people-pleaser; please yourself first.
10. Dress to impress. When you look good, you feel good and your self-esteem is given a boost.

More than 80 percent of African American women are overweight or obese, according to the ***National Institute of Health***. Nearly 12 percent of black women have diabetes, 37 percent have high blood pressure and 48 percent have high cholesterol. Although heart disease is the number one health concern among all Americans, black women are affected at a rate that is an astonishing 72 percent higher than white women. The root cause is linked to excessive weight and lack of exercise. Further studies commissioned by the American Heart Association revealed that although 60 percent of white women were aware of heart disease as the leading cause of death for women, less than half of African American (43 percent), Hispanic (44 percent) and Asian (34 percent) women identified heart disease as the leading cause. In addition, most women lacked knowledge of evidence-based therapies for preventing cardiovascular disease, and half of women aged between 25 and 34 were unaware of heart disease as the number one killer in women's health. This demonstrates the need for prevention education to help avert death and disability from this deadly, yet ultimately preventable, disease.

Test Your Knowledge

The national guideline sets "*normal*" blood pressure at 120/80 but some medical professionals consider that standard to be arbitrary. Some believe your target blood pressure level can be determined only within the context of your other cardiovascular risk factors. For instance, diabetics that have high cholesterol and are overweight would like to see their blood pressure at 110/70 or lower. The concept of "normal" blood pressure is one of the major misconceptions many of us have about hypertension.

If you are among the 73 million Americans who have high blood pressure, how much do you know about your condition? Here are a few things you should know:

TRUE OR FALSE: ***Your cholesterol level matters more than blood pressure.***

Actually, the opposite is often more true. If you have high cholesterol but your ratio of HDL ("good") to LDL ("bad") is healthy or if your cholesterol particles tend to be at large, your risk of a heart attack is not great. High blood pressure puts stress on your blood vessels, including those supplying your heart with blood, and this stress makes it easier for the bad LDL cholesterol particles to penetrate the inner lining of your vessel walls. If allowed to accumulate on the inner lining, a plaque forms that can eventually lead to a heart attack or stroke.

TRUE OR FALSE: ***If you have hypertension, you should measure your blood pressure every day.*** Once a week is often enough to measure your blood pressure. Although a home measuring device helps individuals manage their blood pressure, the monitoring process can effectively lead to an increase in stress levels. However, if your physician instructs you to monitor your pressure daily, please do so. Always follow the doctor's orders! Keep track of your average blood pressure over many months and give that information to your doctor on your next visit. In the same way that it's not advisable, or necessary, to weigh yourself every day to see if you're losing weight, it's not necessary to check your blood pressure every day. Damage occurs over years, not days or weeks so daily checks can be more de-motivating than motivating. You will lose weight and your blood pressure will improve if you simply continue to do the right thing consistently!

TRUE OR FALSE: ***If I'm hypertensive and feel bad, it's probably because my blood pressure has elevated.***

This is almost never the case. Whatever is causing your symptoms is elevating your blood pressure, not the other way around. When you're not feeling well, your body releases adrenaline, causing your blood pressure to elevate.

My Life Check: Live Better with Life's Simple 7

My Life Check was designed by the American Heart Association to help us all live a long, productive, healthy life. Each of us can make small changes in these seven areas that will add up to a big difference in our heart health.

1. Get Active

We suggest at least 150 minutes per week of moderate exercise or 75 minutes per week of vigorous exercise or a combination of moderate and vigorous.

Moderate activity = an activity that elevates your heart and breathing rate above normal levels but you remain comfortable. For example, walking at a moderate pace would make you feel warm and slightly breathless but you would be able to carry on a conversation throughout.

Vigorous activity = an activity that elevates your heart and 'breathing rate to a level that begins to feel uncomfortable and you feel that you are pushing yourself to continue. For example, walking at a vigorous pace would make it difficult for you to carry on a normal conversation as you would be limited to short sentences or just one or two words at a time. Walking can be made an even more vigorous activity by including hilly terrain.

2. Control Cholesterol

A cholesterol level of 200 mg/dL or higher puts you in a high-risk category and is cause to take action. The first steps toward lowering high cholesterol levels are to exercise regularly and eat a healthy diet. This means cutting down on trans fats in your diet and replacing unhealthy saturated fats with healthier unsaturated alternatives. There is also scientific evidence to support the belief that eating certain foods can also help to lower cholesterol, including garlic, soya and oats.

3. Eat Better

Vegetables and fruits are high in vitamins, minerals and fiber□and they're low in calories. Eating a variety of fruits and vegetables may help you control your weight and your blood pressure.

4. Manage Blood Pressure

Good news! High blood pressure is manageable. Even if your blood pressure is normal (less than 120 mm Hg systolic AND less than 80 mm Hg diastolic) and your goal is prevention only, the lifestyle modifications outlined here provide a prescription for healthy living.

5. Lose Weight

Among Americans aged 20 years and older, 145 million are overweight or obese (BMI of 25.0 kg/m2 and higher). That's 76.9 million men and 68.1 million women. This is of great concern, especially since obesity is now recognized as a major, independent risk factor for heart disease. If you have too much fat—especially if a lot of it is at your waist—you're at higher risk for such health problems as high blood pressure, high blood cholesterol and diabetes.

6. Reduce Blood Sugar

When diabetes is detected, a doctor may prescribe changes in eating habits, weight control, exercise programs and medication to keep it in check. It's critical for people with diabetes to have regular check-ups. Work closely with your healthcare provider to manage your diabetes and control any other risk factors. For example, blood pressure for people with diabetes should be lower than 130/80 mm Hg.

7. Stop Smoking

Smoking by itself increases the risk of coronary heart disease. When it acts with the other factors, it greatly increases your risk from those factors too. Smoking decreases your tolerance for physical activity and decreases your HDL (good) cholesterol levels. It also increases the tendency for your blood to clot so if you smoke and have a family history of heart disease, you greatly increase your own risks.

Not all forms of exercise are suitable for all people but that in no way rules out all forms of exercise! Your current size or underlying health problems may make certain activities unsuitable or unadvisable for you but there are *always* alternatives. For example, if you have a heart condition, floor exercises must be avoided as they can cause problems with blood flow to and from the heart but a traditional exercise such as a push-up can be performed just as effectively standing up and pushing against a wall instead of the floor.

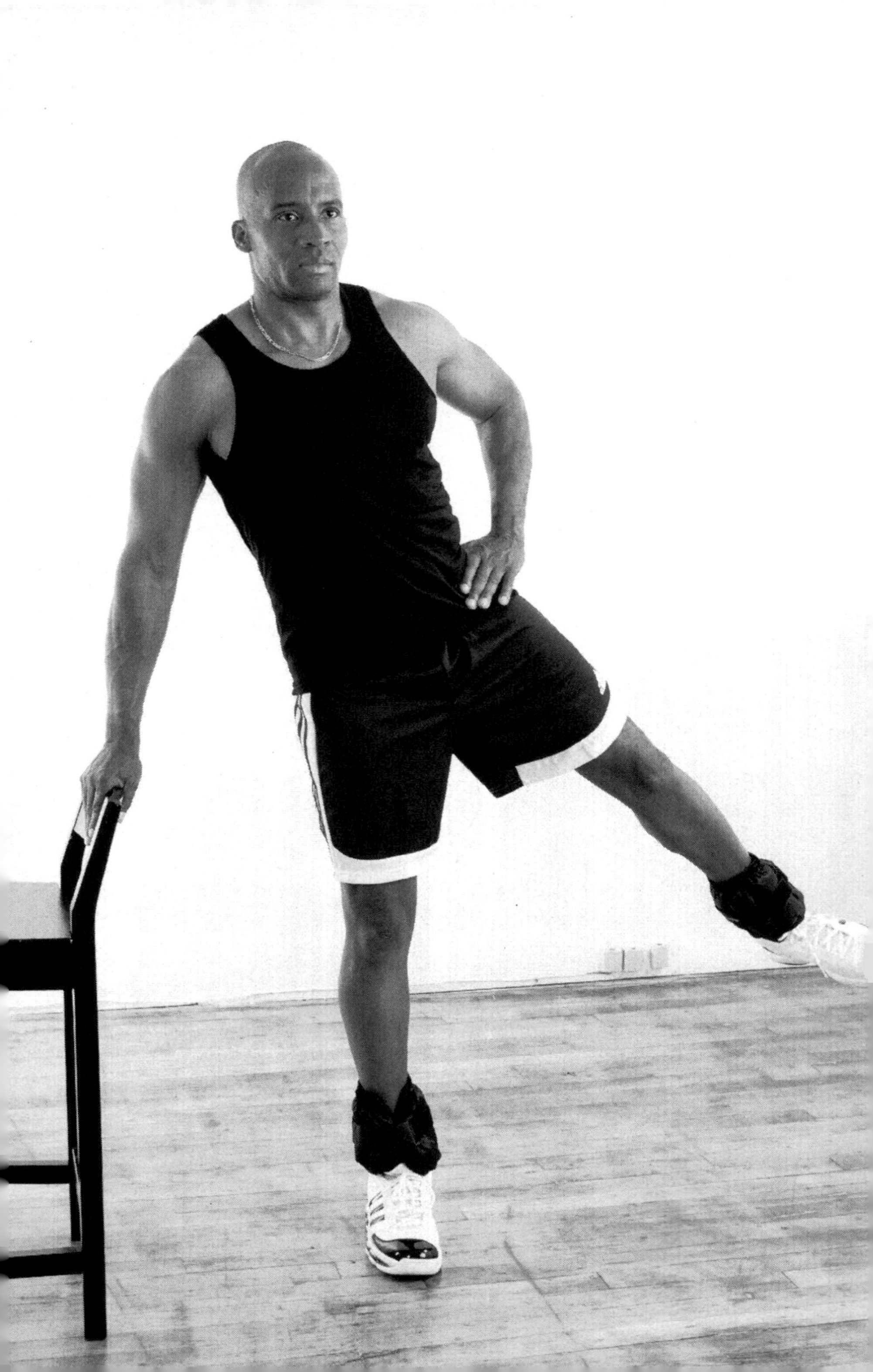

Chapter 8
Lose While You Snooze

"Sometimes the most urgent thing you can possibly do is take a complete rest."

- Ashleigh Brilliant

Do you believe that being healthy involves good nutrition, cardiovascular training and strength training only? That's far from the truth. Getting proper rest is of equal importance and essential to leading a full and healthy life.

One sure way to drop some excess pounds is to give your body the rest it needs.

Getting at least 7.5 to 8 hours of sleep every night has been proven to enhance your life in many ways. While it may be obvious that sleep is beneficial, most people don't realize how much sleep they really need and why it is so important to get it. According to ***The Division of Sleep Medicine at Harvard Medical School***, your body manages and requires sleep in much the same way that it regulates the need for eating, drinking and breathing. Extensive research has been carried out on the effects of sleep and the studies have consistently shown that sleep plays a vital role in promoting physical health, longevity of life and emotional well-being.

The results of studies have also shown that people who get fewer hours of sleep per night tend to weigh more. Sanjay Patel, M.D.A., researcher at *Western Reserve University in Cleveland*, found that those who slept five or less hours per night were 30 percent more likely to gain 30-plus pounds than those who got more rest. Our body needs sleep so that it can rebuild lean muscle mass which allows us to burn more fat, even as we rest. Some experts believe that lack of sleep is one reason for America's obesity epidemic. Individuals who get fewer hours of sleep per night tend to weigh more. The National Sleep Foundation found that the average woman gets six hours and 40 minutes of sleep most nights but many people are sleep deprived for various reasons, including hectic work schedules, family responsibilities and stress. When our bodies are under stress we release a stress hormone called cortisol which throws our body off balance. This can not only result in weight gain, but other physical and psychological issues also. That is why stress management techniques are important and useful to all of us before "calling it a night."

A Good Night's Sleep Will—

- •Rejuvenate your mind and body, and prepare you for the next day.
- •Help your body rebuild lean muscle mass after a good weight training workout and burn calories while you sleep.
- Help heal tired and sore muscles from daily activities.
- Help regulate your metabolic rate which will help burn fat.

Getting Quality "Z's"

Now that we have listed some ways that sleep can help your body lose weight, here are some practical ways of helping yourself to get some quality Z's!

- **Room Décor**

The way your room is arranged is very important in terms of helping you to achieve quality sleep. Make sure you have relaxing colors, such as light green, baby blue or other relaxing colors that make you feel calm.

Also, be sure to have a comfortable comforter, bed sheets, blankets and bed sheets. Lighting should be dim when you are about to fall asleep and a clean, clutter-free environment is also more relaxing. Air quality and circulation is important for your breathing so a humidifier may be helpful in some climates, and a cooler room is more comfortable than a room that becomes too hot. If you begin to sweat throughout the night, your sleep will be interrupted so it's important to find a temperature that's comfortable for you. It's also advisable to avoid having the TV on when trying to fall asleep as this can prevent you from reaching 'stage 3' of the sleep cycle. (Details of the 5 Stages of Sleep can be found below).

- **Meditation Techniques**

When we take time to meditate or do some deep breathing exercises, this helps to relax both body and mind, and also relieve stress. Individuals who practice meditation tend to have a lower resting heart rate, meaning the heart works less strenuously to pump blood throughout the body. Along with creating a potential drop in cholesterol levels, there can also be a reduction of free radicals—unstable oxygen molecules that cause tissue damage within the body. A decrease in the number of free radicals is important because they play an integral role in the aging process. It's thought that if we could slow down or eliminate the proliferation of free radicals, we may actually be able to slow the aging process!

Tip: Try to set aside five to 15 minutes a few times a week to meditate. I find taking a bath is a "2 for 1" way to relax my body and mind.

- **Warm Bath**

A warm bath with Epsom or bath salts will help you relax and prepare you for a good night's sleep. I suggest doing this at least three times a week. Try burning some candles and relax for at least 20 minutes; this is one of the best ways to prepare your body and mind for relaxation.

- **Brainstorming**

A busy mind is a guaranteed way to toss and turn, and ultimately lose sleep. A good way to help release those clustered thoughts is to grab a pen and pad to write them down. Writing your thoughts down will help you sub-consciously relieve stress and rest throughout the night.

- **Reading**

Reading a good book is always a great relaxing tool to help ease the mind and shift your body into relaxation mode. Reading an inspirational book is one of my favorite ways to end my day on a positive note—and let me tell you, it's better than the 11 o'clock news!

- **Soft Music**

Inspirational or mellow music is always a good recipe to help you fall asleep. Also, you can use natural sound effects such as rain and waterfall CDs to create a tranquil environment.

- **Eat Right**

Try to avoid eating heavy meals within two hours before turning in for the night. A heavy meal in your stomach before you go to bed will cause your body to lose quality sleep as the digestive system continues to work overtime throughout the night in an effort to digest your food. If you must eat a meal before you go to bed, make sure it is a light one such as soup or a salad. Protein based foods are the better choice because the protein content will help to repair any damaged muscle and aid the rebuilding process. Going to bed hungry will also disturb your sleep but at all costs, avoid all caffeinated drinks before going to bed.

- **Herbal Tea**

Chamomile and "Sleepytime" tea is a good way to unwind after a long hard day. A cup of hot tea before going to bed will soothe your body and help you rest.

The 5 Stages of Sleep
(Based on information from the Stanford Sleep Book)

Stage 1 – we enter the transition state as we fall asleep and begin our first "sleep cycle." This light sleep stage lasts from 2-5 minutes and if sleep remains uninterrupted it will progress to stage 2 sleep. Stage 1 gives 2-5% of normal sleep.

Stage 2 – is a much deeper sleep than stage 1. The brain waves go into theta mode, and leads into stages 3 and 4 in about 10-20 minutes. Stage 2 sleep occupies approximately 50-65% of our sleep time, lasting 15-30 minutes in each cycle. During the second part of the night we spend more and more time alternating between stages 2 & REM sleep.

Stage 3 – is a much deeper sleep than stage 2. The muscles are relaxed, the heart rate slows down, the blood pressure falls, and the breathing is steady and even. Brain activity slows down noticeably from the theta pattern of stage 2 to a much slower rhythm of 1 to 2 cycles per second called delta sleep system, and the height or amplitude of the waves increase.
Stage 4 – is the deepest sleep of all, during which a sleeping person is "dead to the world." Blood pressure and heart rate change and the sleeper's brain heats ups. The delta sleep system is characterized by very high voltage, slow brain waves.

<u>Stage 5 REM</u> (rapid eye movement) – the first REM period lasts only about 10 minutes. After that, the sleeper goes back into a deep stage 4 sleep or the delta sleep system. Again, the sleeper returns into a REM stage after a short period and cycles through REM stage 4 continue until the sleeper wakes up.

It has been proven that making the simple changes listed above can not only help you "lose while you snooze" by aiding weight loss, it can also help you to live longer.

Sign Me Up!

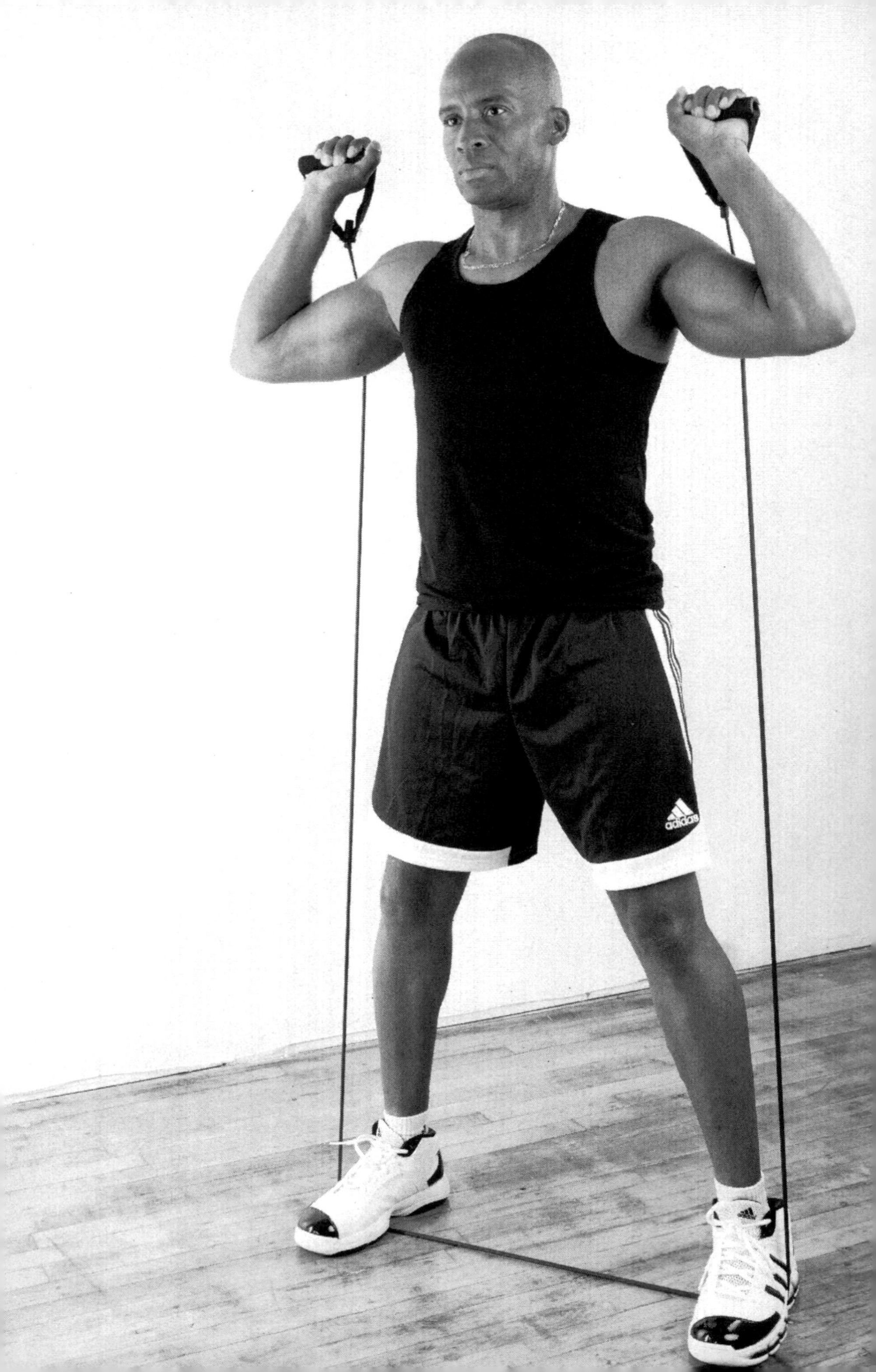
adidas

Chapter 9

Good Hair versus Bad Health

"Don't remove the kinks from your hair, remove them from your brain!"
- Marcus Gravey

I have been a personal trainer for more than a decade, and one of the biggest concerns among my female clients has been **HAIR** – they want to know how working out and sculpting their bodies can be possible ***without*** destroying their hair. This is a legitimate concern because I realize that going to the hair salon two or three times a week is not only expensive, it is also unrealistic, especially if you work in Corporate America. We have been conditioned to believe that women with straight, long hair are more appealing in the business arena than those who have a natural hair style. Of course, it is my personal opinion that wearing a natural hairstyle is not only attractive, it's great for working out because it's stress free and low maintenance. However, there is no denying that first impressions matter in all areas of life, so looking the part is very important. With that said, many women, especially African American women, have a dilemma. What comes first – good hair or good health? I witness so many ladies with slammin' hairstyles, manicured nails, and eloquent business suits—who are overweight and unhealthy. What sense does that make? Why have nice-looking nails, a fresh hairstyle and be dressed to the "9s" yet subtract 10 to 15 years off your life because of obesity and heart disease?

Beauty starts from the inside out and I believe that all women can have great hair *AND* a healthy body to match.

I can say this with authority because so many of my clients are professional women who are doctors, lawyers, business owners and housewives who have found the secret to physical and cosmetic wholeness. It *is* possible to look the part corporately and still have sex appeal on your fitness journey. So, let's spend some time discussing some ways we can make this happen. Even if you are one of those fortunate women who has hair that doesn't require a lot of maintenance, you can still learn some tips about exercising while maintaining a good hairstyle.

I interviewed one of my long-time friends and clients who is a hairstylist with over 20 years of experience. She is a wife, mother, weight trainer and marathon runner who has discovered the secret to having good hair and total health. Michelle Watson is a hairstylist at Sheer Joy Hair Studio located in Owings Mills, MD. She works demanding hours, but still finds time to weight train at least three times a week. Recently, I asked her to reveal how she can manage to juggle so much – and all without having a "*bad hair day.*" Here is her response—

> *"The foundation to having fitness ready hair style and still maintain a nice professional look begins with a haircut. With a great cut you are able to maintain a decent look even after a tough workout. Keeping the hair regularly conditioned is also a key factor, since the excessive salt we produce through working out can be very drying to the hair and can lead*

to other adverse results to relaxed hair overtime. For those who opt to change their look with extensions, your options are extensive ranging through different textures from curly, straight, wavy lengths and color."

In the hair world today, there are many options to choose from. There really is no excuse if you desire to change your body and still maintain a great hairstyle—a healthy hairstyle! All it takes is a little creativity and planning to get started. If you are serious about your health and wellness there are plenty of options available to make it happen. Women of other ethnic groups can run, jump and lift weights, then head to the locker room, wash their hair, blow dry it and continue on with their day – all without missing a beat. That's just how it is! African American women may have a slight disadvantage compared to women of other cultures because of the texture of their hair, but this doesn't give you a reason not to take care of your health. It may mean that you have to work a little harder and do a little more, but the benefits are endless. Think of it this way; your family and friends are counting on you to live a long and healthy life without heart disease, diabetes, cancer and obesity. You mean way too much to way too many people to allow cosmetic issues to shorten your pre-destined destiny. My mission is to rescue as many women as possible in order to keep our communities strong, healthy, and productive.

Healthy Hair

Listed below are a few hairstyle alternatives that can provide practical ways to have great health and great hair:

- **Sport Cut**

Have your stylist design a cut that is conducive to your gym time, professional career and social life. You may have to have your hair trimmed more often than normal, but with regular maintenance you can have beautiful, healthy hair. If finances are an issue, you may have to cut back on a few lattés and other such luxuries to make this happen, but the right cut will take you a long way.

- **Braids**

The good news is that braids will lasts up to six weeks before you have to get new ones. Having your hair braided gives you the opportunity to sweat hard, then wash and go. I have seen this approach being used more often in gyms across America, simply because it's low maintenance and a great money saver. The micro-mini braids are a good choice because they will give you the option to go straight, sport a pony-tail, or pin your hair up. Good move ladies!

- **Hair Weave**

A nice weave is good because it will last a little longer than braids, but it has to be a good one. You may have to spend a little more on the front end, but it will be worth it in the long-run. With a good weave you can work out with pony-tail and still look good at your Monday morning business meeting. Not only will you get compliments on your hair, your arms and shoulders will catch everyone's attention too.

- **Wigs**

Maybe it's me, but I find it sometimes impossible to tell the difference between a wig and real hair! With a wig, you can get away with so much, and a woman can choose any hairstyle she wants instantly. Even if your hair is a hot mess after one of my intense workout sessions, you can go to the locker room and transform yourself in less than 30 minutes.

- **The Natural Look**

Wearing your hair natural is a look that only a few women can pull off! You have to have a certain swagger to make this hairstyle work for you, but Jill Scott, Lauren Hill, and India Arie are great examples of women who have successfully made their natural hairstyle look classy and sophisticated. You may feel that a natural look works well in the entertainment world, but not in the business arena—and you may be right. But, it is a hairstyle that will definitely work well with exercise and fit your lifestyle, so why not give it a try? I am almost sure you won't get demoted or lose your job!

- **Pony-Tail**

Sporting a pony-tail is the classic gym and aerobic look. A pony-tail will allow you to enjoy your workout without having your hair getting in the way. So bring on the sweat and let it dry.

Hair Maintenance

You may choose to take the options listed above for various reasons or you may already be comfortable exercising with your current hairstyle. However, the following tips will help you manage your hair through even the most vigorous aerobics class, outdoor run, yoga routine, or strength training program. These tips have all been tried, tested and proven to help women preserve their hairstyle until the next hair appointment.

Three Tips to Use While Working Out:

1. Head Band

Wearing a head band will help absorb most of your sweat while you exercise. Also, it will allow your hair to breathe without having your head completely covered. I know it's the Jane Fonda look from the 70s, but it still works – and now the head bands are much cuter than the ones from the 70s!

2. Head Scarf

Unlike a head band, a head scarf will completely cover your head and absorb more sweat. This is an advantage if you have a short haircut and it will also help your hair stay in place once it has completely dried.

3. Hair Pins

Some of my clients who have longer hair will take the time to pin their hair up before taking a group fitness class. This may take longer, but it will allow your hair to breathe while you exercise and sweat. Once you get home, you can simply remove the hair pins and let your hair dry naturally.

Now that hair is no longer an issue because you can—
Wrap it, pin it, extend it, braid it, cover it, cut it or shake it –
Go ahead and do what whatever it takes to get your body in shape!

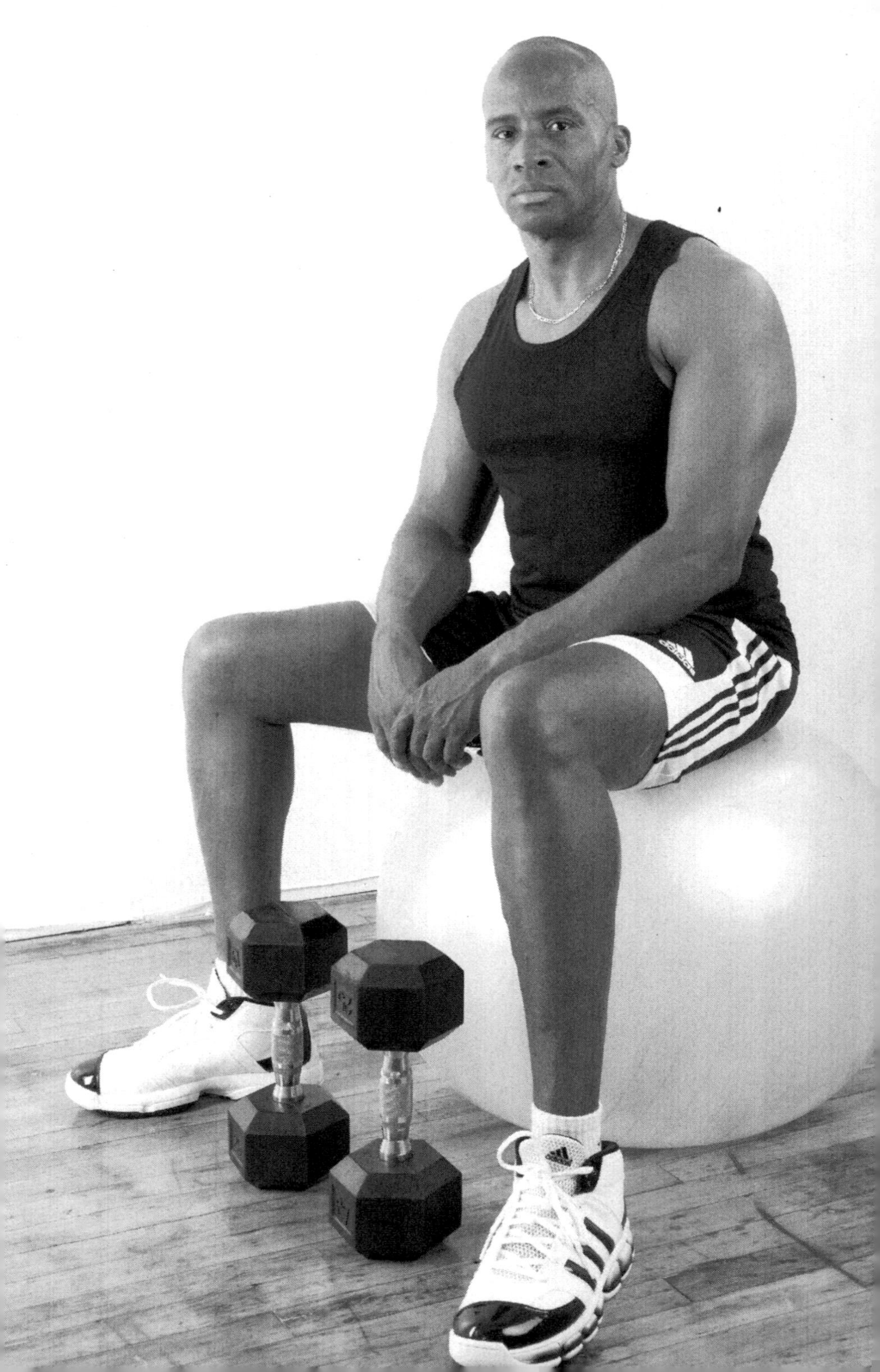

Chapter 10

The "I'm Too Cute to Sweat" 21 Day Workout

First of all, I would like to take the opportunity to applaud all you women out there for the outstanding job you do every day as mothers, teachers, and business professionals. The list goes on. Women wear so many hats and do so many things – that's why the world is a better place with you in it! So, it is very important that you should take time for yourself, because you always give so much of yourself to others.

As I stated earlier, cardiovascular disease is the number one killer among women. Several reasons for this are bad eating habits, lack of exercise, being overweight and stress. My 21 Day Workout will not only help you to get into fitness mode, it will complement whatever exercise program you are currently doing. You will not have to alter your schedule at all as this routine is designed to fit perfectly into your everyday lifestyle. You will be amazed by how much better you feel and look in the first 21 days, and this program is geared to help women of all fitness levels. The key to success, as with any other program, is to start – and remain – consistent. You are already doing most of these movements naturally but before we get to the hands-on routine, there are three important elements that must be in place. These elements are things you may already be doing but if not, they are easy to begin and by getting into the habit of doing them, you will help yourself to achieve the results you want much faster. The objective for the next 21 days is to help you reach your full potential by providing you with a stronger, faster and healthier body. **You must do the following for 21 days straight!** Consistency is the key to this program.

Three Crucial Elements

1. **Drink at least 8 ounces of water first thing in the morning.**

Drinking water will help hydrate you and provide your body with the necessary nutrients to start your day. Water is your body's most important nutrient; it is involved in every bodily function, and makes up 70-75 percent of your total body weight. Water helps you to maintain body temperature and metabolize body fat; it also aids in digestion, lubricates and cushions organs, transports nutrients and flushes toxins from your body. Everyone should drink at least 64 ounces of water per day, and if you exercise or are overweight, even more. Your blood is approximately 90 percent water and is responsible for transporting nutrients and energy to muscles and for taking waste from tissues. If you are not getting enough water, your body will react by pulling it from other places, including your blood. This causes the closing of some smaller vessels (capillaries), making your blood thicker, more susceptible to clotting and harder to pump through your system which can have serious implications, not least hypertension, high cholesterol and heart disease. Recent studies have also linked a lack of proper hydration to headaches, arthritis and heartburn. Have you ever gotten up in the morning feeling bloated; or tried on a ring or shoe that fit just fine yesterday but is too tight to wear today? If you have, the chances are your body is trying to tell you something. If you have a problem with water retention, excess salt may be the cause. Your body will tolerate a certain amount of sodium, however, the more salt you consume, the more fluid you need to dilute it. To overcome this

problem, always drink plenty of water.
Tip: Buy a case of water and place it in your bedroom or bathroom.

2. **Write it down.**

Before I start any work out plan with new clients, the first thing that I have them do is some positive self-talk. We all have a little voice in our heads that says something like, "I can't lose weight," or, "I don't have time to exercise." The minute we start verbalizing our negative thoughts, we automatically set ourselves up for failure. One way to overcome negative thoughts and negative self-talk is to learn the power of positive affirmations. We need to pay more attention to our thought process in all areas of life and this holds true in exercise. Each time your inner voice starts saying words such as "can't" or fills your mind with negative thoughts such as "what if I can't do it; what if I fail?" or "what if I just make a fool of myself; what if I get hurt; what if I just end up looking the same but with bad hair?" you need to verbally overcome those thoughts with positive self-talk in the form of positive affirmations.

Positive affirmations are the foundations to achieving our physical, spiritual, and mental goals. For example; if you want to lose 10 pounds in 30 days, say, "I am losing 10 pounds in 30 days"! Every word you speak, whether positive or negative, has a major impact on your life. Your focus must always be positive and your affirmations must reflect your positive attitude. There are going to be times when you feel bad physically or feel "down" emotionally but you must continue to believe in yourself as the person you are striving to become. Never give in to negative thoughts and answer back to your negative voice by saying words like, "I feel young healthy and strong; I have never felt better than I to do right now," or, "by His stripes I am healed!"

You *are* who you say you are in your positive affirmations and you *can* do what you say you can!

Life and death is in the power of the tongue. On an index card, write out your desired mission for the next 21 days and where you would like to be at the end of that time period. Your goals will have to go beyond your emotions because your feelings are so unpredictable; one day you're feeling up and the next day you may be feeling down. Your language over the next three weeks will make or break you. Positive affirmation will be your secret weapon for your 21 day journey! Throughout the day, every day, verbally say what you **want – not** what you **don't want**. No matter how you *perceive* things to be, start speaking good health into your life right now! Once you condition your words, your body will take you exactly where it needs to go and show you how to get there. Clarity is power. Tell yourself, and therefore your body, exactly what you want to achieve and how you want to look. In so doing, you create a powerful "why" to remind yourself of your reasons why you're doing what you're doing. Your reasons will come before your answers and your "why" has to be bigger than your "can't". You may have to find a bigger reason than simply looking good to help push through those days when you feel like giving up.

Say What You Mean, Mean What You Say

Enthusiasm comes from within and when you have it, you are sure to win. Here are some examples of phrases you can use to help boost your motivation and keep you going through the process of change over the next 21 days.

I feel like a teenager again!
These pounds are dropping off like water!
This is the strongest I have felt in my life!
My energy level is out of control!
I have never felt better than I do right now!
This is the healthiest I have been in my entire life!
Everywhere I go these days, I light up the room!
My body is full of so much power!
I really love the person that I'm becoming!
I am blessed and highly favored!
I'm wonderfully and fearfully made!

By doing this simple exercise, you will train your body to do what you want. Just reading the list of phrases makes you feel good! Now add at least 10 of your own phases. Don't be modest!

1. ____
2. ____
3. ____
4. ____
5. ____
6. ____
7. ____
8. ____
9. ____
10. ____

Tip: Place your card on your bathroom mirror or on the seat of your car, somewhere highly visible on a daily basis.

3. Eat fruit at least once every day!

Fruits have natural nutrients that processed foods cannot provide. A piece of fruit is a great way to start off your day because your body needs the carbohydrates for energy and brain function. Fruit is the ideal food for exercise. In fact, the best post-workout snack or meal is not muffins, yogurt, or protein shakes, but fresh fruit. Runners and other athletes have long known that there is nothing better than high-water content, sweet fruit, such as oranges or melons, after a workout. They contain enough water to hydrate the body and their natural sugars are quickly utilized for energy production. If your sole purpose in terms of diet and exercise is fat loss, you should never eat a carbohydrate alone and should include a protein and an essential fatty acid in your snack or meal along with your carbohydrate. Regular physical activity improves insulin sensitivity, which is the effectiveness of insulin in transporting sugar to your cells. In other words, if you exercise, you will be able to utilize fruit sugar a lot better and will be less likely to experience "sugar swings" and blood sugar fluctuations. This is one area most people miss because of all the fast food and unhealthy snack options out there.

Tip: Keep a bowl of fresh fruit on your kitchen table to remind you to grab a piece in the morning.

What You Need

Do you know where to find the best fitness center in America? I will tell you – your home! This is the one place where don't have to worry about how you look, what you have on, how your make up looks, or whether or not you have brushed your teeth. At home you can be you. You won't have to worry about someone looking at you, pushing up on you or asking for your number. However, it would be helpful to have the following pieces of equipment if available. These items are not mandatory but you may wish to consider purchasing them soon.

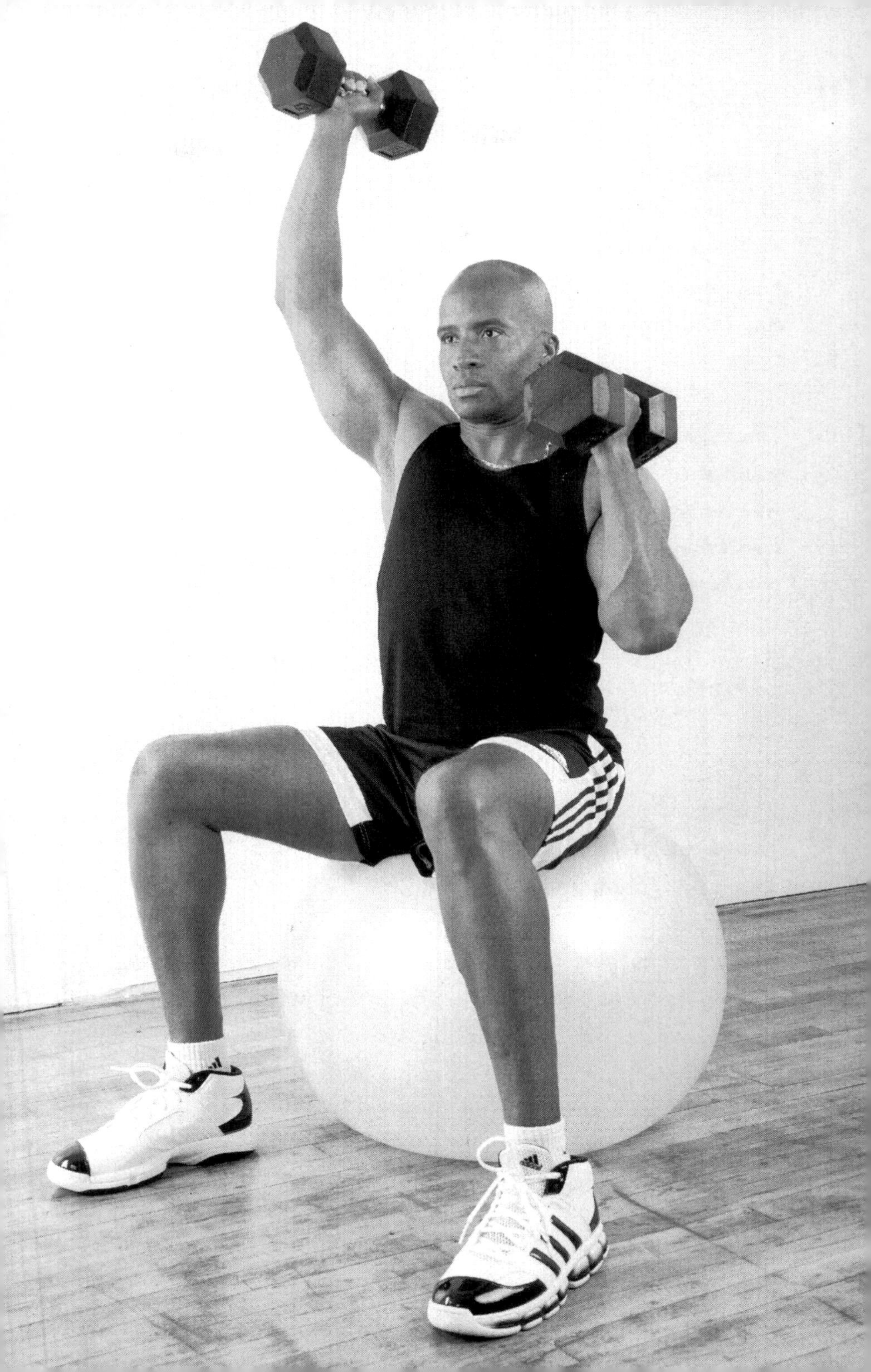

- **Two hand weights of 3-5 pounds**
- **Two hand weights of 10-15 pounds**
- **A set of 5-10 pounds ankle weights**
- **A stability fitness ball**
- **A resistance workout band**

Let's Get Physical!

This is your time to transform yourself with peace of mind. I will help you make each room of your home a gym. Just designate each room of your home to focus on a particular body part and you will have your very own world class fitness center in your very own home—with a lifetime membership!

Too Cute to Sweat Exercise 1
Bathroom Shoulder Press

Equipment: All you need is your commode and a pair of 10-15 pounds weights.

Target Area: Shoulders and triceps

Exercise:

• Place a pair of 10-15 pounds weights next to the commode.

• When sitting on the commode, pick up your weights and hold them at shoulder height with your wrists facing forward.

• Lift the weights up above your head by straightening your arms, being careful not to hyper extend your elbows—keep your elbow joints relaxed—then lower the weights slowly back down to shoulder height ready to repeat the exercise.

Repetitions: Every time you enter the bathroom you should do at least

15 repetitions (reps), ideally two sets of 15 reps with a short rest in between sets. Even if you are not actually using the restroom, place the commode lid down and work your shoulders.

Too Cute to Sweat Exercise 2
Ankle Weights

Equipment: A set of 5-10 pounds ankle weights.
Target Area: Leg and glutes muscles
Exercise:
Simply wear your ankle weights around your home as you carry on with your regular routine. Aim to spend at least 15-45 minutes each day wearing your weights; add front and side leg raises to increase the intensity of the exercise.
Front leg Raises:
• In a standing position, shift your weight on to one leg so that you can raise the other leg slightly from the floor. Keep good posture in your upper body.
• Keeping the raised leg straight at the knee, raise it out in front of you—a few more inches from the ground is all it takes.
• Pause for a few seconds at the highest point before slowly returning your leg to the starting position ready to repeat the exercise without allowing your foot to return to the floor.
• Aim to complete 15 reps before switching legs to repeat the exercise.
Side leg Raises:
• Begin in the same starting position as the front leg raises exercise.
• Keeping the raised leg straight at the knee, move it away from your body out to the side—again, a raise of just a few inches is all it takes.

• Be careful to maintain an upright posture in your upper body and avoid leaning over to the side or bending your spine as you raise your leg.
• Pause for a second or two at the highest point and then slowly return to the starting position without allowing your foot to touch the floor.
• Aim to complete 15 reps on each leg.

Tip: Lean against the wall or hold onto a piece of solid furniture to aid your balance as you perform the leg raises. These exercises help tone the front of your legs and hips and when you remove the ankle weights, you will definitely feel a big difference in your legs.

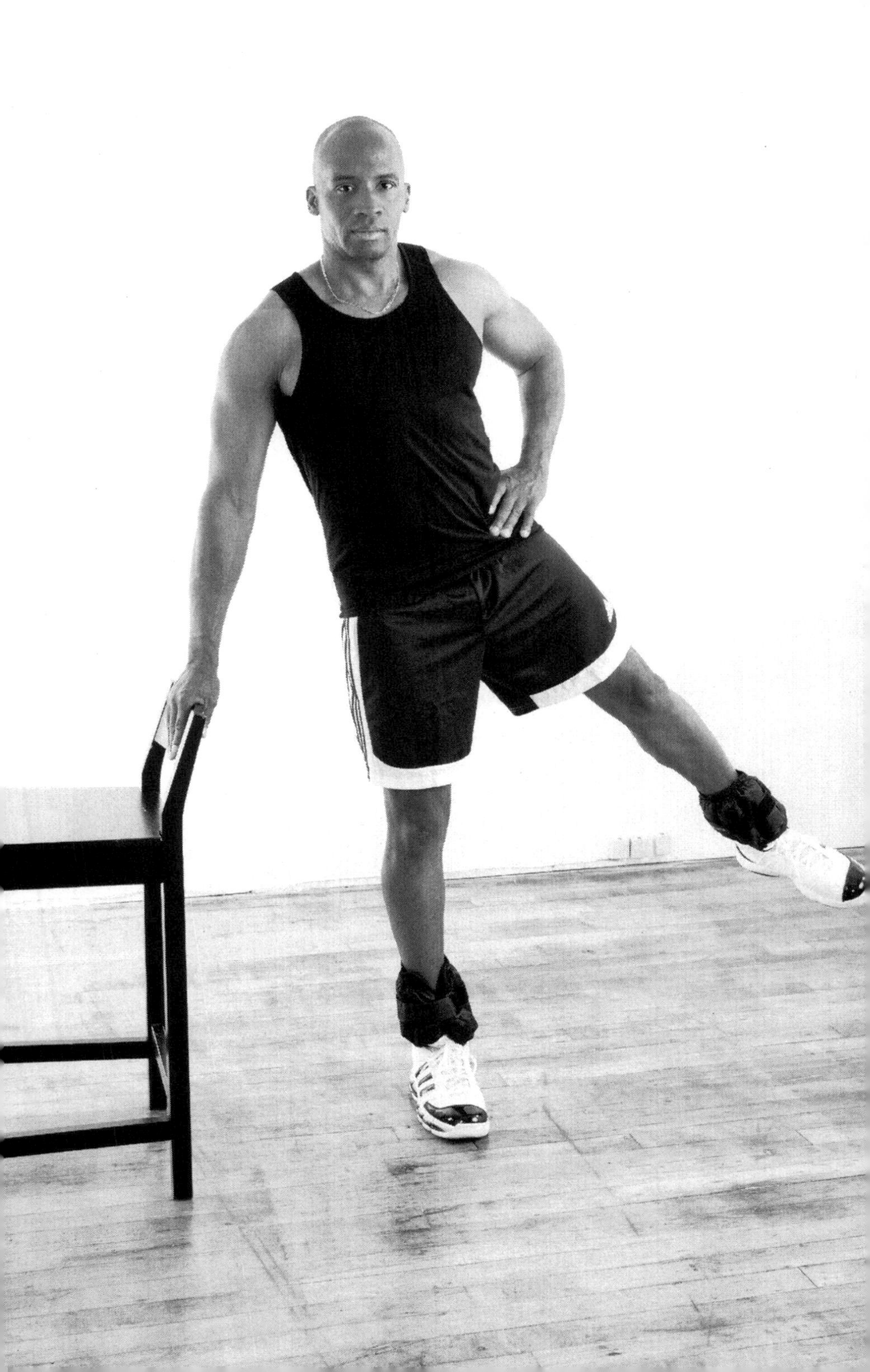

Too Cute to Sweat Exercise 3
Kitchen Workout

Equipment: A pair of 3-5 pounds weights
Target Area: Shoulders and arm muscles
Exercise:

When you go to the kitchen to get a snack, use your 5 pounds weights to do some lateral raises with your arms.

Lateral Raises:

• Begin with a weight in each hand and your arms relaxed by your sides.

• Keeping your arms straight, but with elbow joints relaxed, slowly raise your arms up and away from your body until the weights reach around shoulder height.

• Pause for a couple of seconds at the top of the raise and then slowly return your arms to the starting position ready to repeat the exercise.

Repetitions: Aim to complete 25 repetitions and build up to doing three sets of 25-30 reps with a short rest between sets.

You can also combine this exercise with front raises, which will define the front of your shoulders. The slower you do these exercises, the better the effect and it's a great way to build and tone your shoulder muscles while giving great definition to your arms.

Front Raises:

• Begin with the weights held to the front of your body with your wrists facing inward toward your thighs.

• Keeping your arms straight with elbows relaxed, raise the weights up and away from your body until they reach around shoulder height.

• Pause at the top before slowly returning to the starting position. The weights should remain shoulder width apart throughout the exercise.

Tip: A great time to do this is when you are placing something in the microwave, using the blender, or preparing dinner. You're standing there anyway, so why not do something to benefit your health while there!

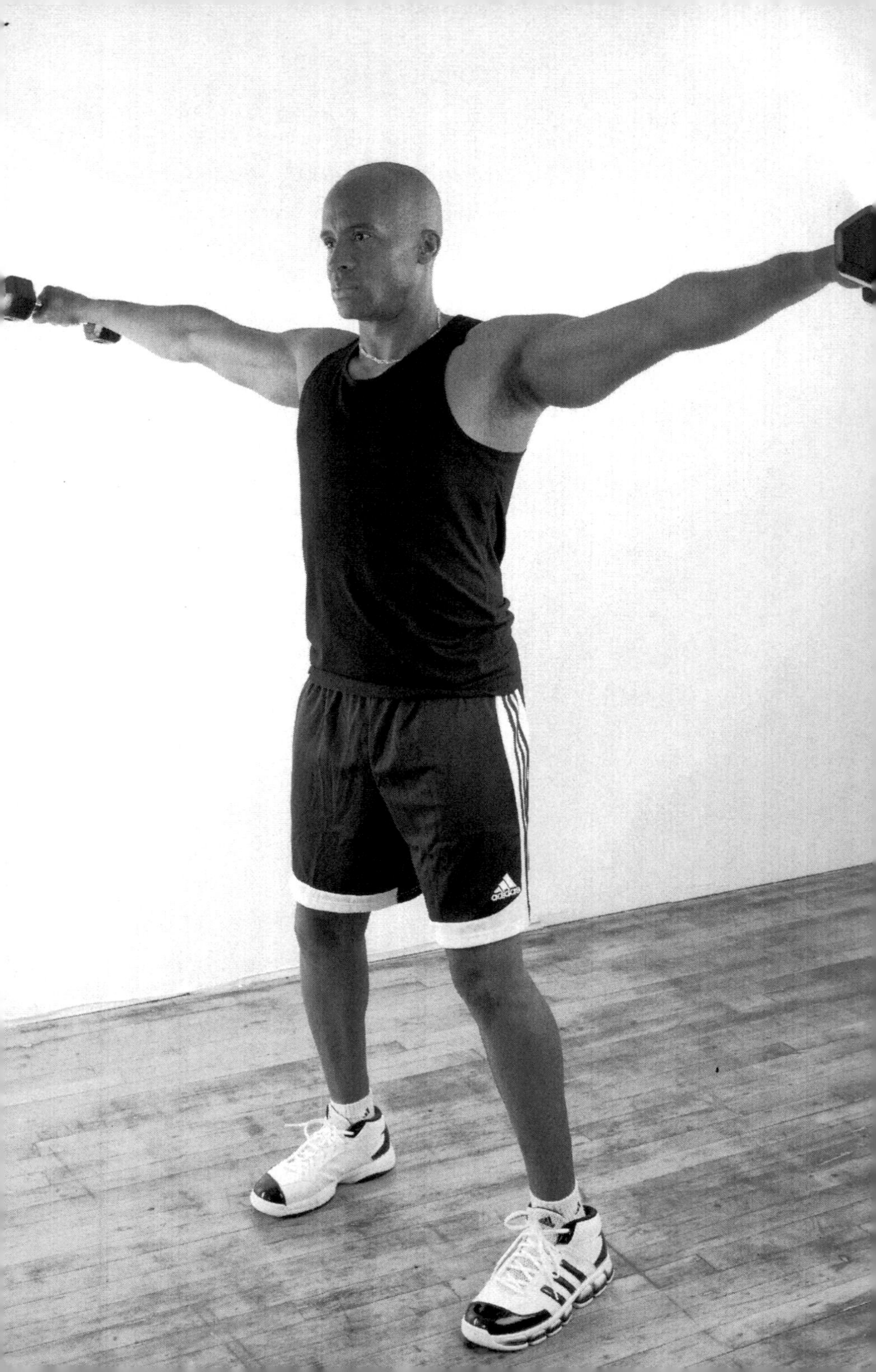

Too Cute to Sweat Exercise 4
Living or Bedroom Resistance Band Workout

Equipment: A pair of resistance bands.
Target Area: Total body
Exercise:
Place your resistance bands in the room where you spend the most time. While watching TV, you can use the resistance bands in between commercial breaks for a good total body workout.
• In a standing position, with feet placed around hip width apart, step on your bands so that one end of each one is fixed in position under each foot.
• Holding the loose end of each band firmly, stretch them out beyond shoulder width.
• Pull the bands behind your shoulders and position your hands at shoulder height with wrists facing forward as if about to do a shoulder press.
• Keeping your arms and hands in the above position, slowly squat down by bending your knees, as if about to sit on a chair.
• Make sure you keep good posture in your upper body as you squat, avoid arching or rounding your spine.
• From the squat position, slowly stand up and push the bands above your head in a shoulder press movement at the same time.
• Return your hands to your shoulders, ready to repeat the exercise.
Repetitions: Aim to complete 15 repetitions and build up to three sets of 15 reps with a short rest between sets. By keeping your resistance bands in the room you spend most time in, this exercise will become the one you do most frequently in the program.

This exercise will work your gluteus maximus (your butt) and all of your leg muscles as well as your upper body at the same time.

Tip: You can also use the resistance bands to do lateral raises and front raises (kitchen workout) to work your shoulders and bicep curls to work the front of your upper arms.

Bicep Curls:

- Stand on your bands to fix them in position as in the above exercise.
- Holding the bands, allow your arms to hang by your sides with wrists facing forward.
- Keeping your upper arm in position, bend your elbows to 'curl' your lower arm toward your upper arm - as if your elbows are pinned to your sides and you are aiming to raise your wrists to meet your shoulders.
- Slowly return your arms to the starting position ready to repeat the exercise.

Repetitions: Aim to complete 25 repetitions and build up to three sets of 25-30 reps with a short rest between sets.

Tip: The shorter the length of the resistance band, the greater the resistance so experiment with how long or short you hold the band to give your body a new challenge.

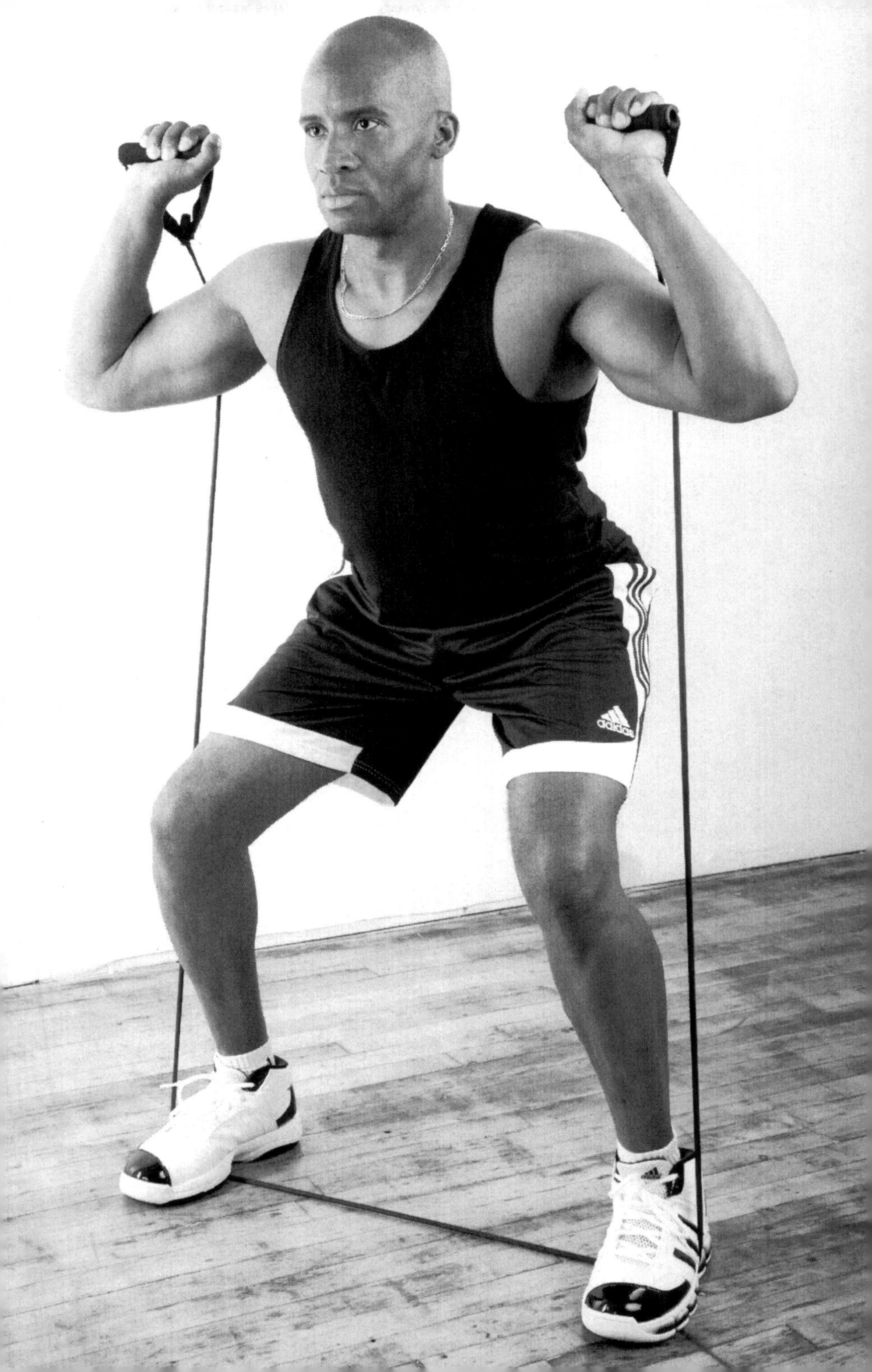
adidas

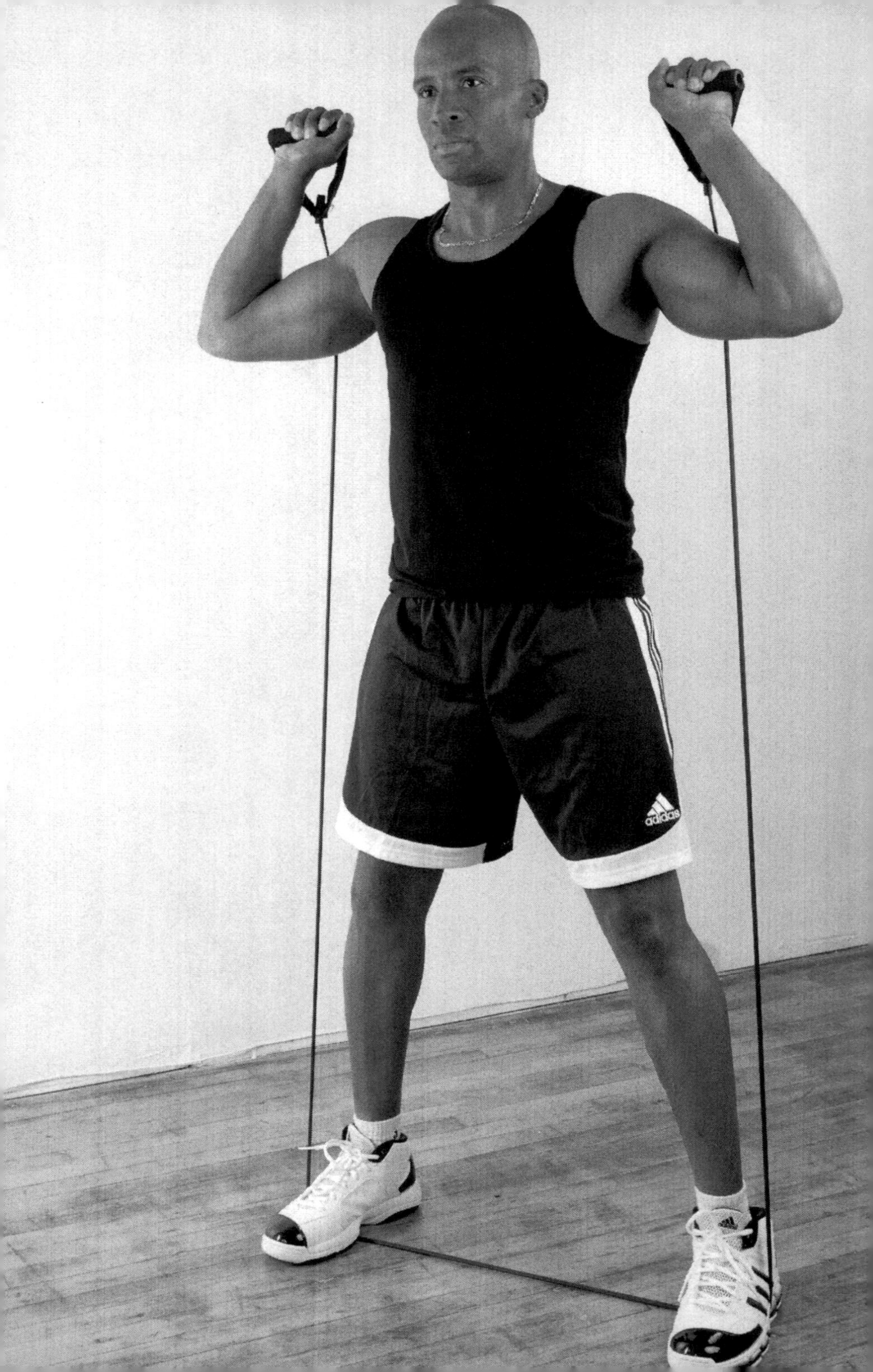
adidas

Too Cute to Sweat Exercise 5
Living Room Ball or Floor Crunches

Equipment: All you need is some floor space or a stability ball if you have one.

Target Area: Abdominal muscles

Exercise:

There are many variations of abdominal crunch exercises so some expert advice from a fitness trainer may be the best way to find the best exercises for you. The following is a basic crunch.

• Position yourself on your back on the floor with your knees bent and the soles of your feet on the floor.

• Place your fingers on your head by your ears.

• Slowly 'crunch' your tummy to raise your shoulders an inch or two from the floor. It's important to protect your neck muscles by keeping a gap between your chin and your chest—as if holding an orange in position under your chin—and avoiding any pull on your head with your fingers.

• Breathe out as you crunch up and breathe in again as you slowly return to the floor, ready to repeat the exercise.

• With practice, you will be able to repeat the exercise without allowing your shoulders to return completely to the floor between crunches. This increases the intensity and the effectiveness of the abdominal crunch exercise.

Repetitions: Every evening before going to bed do 50-100 crunches. Throughout the day when you enter your bedroom, do 25 crunches on a stability ball or on the floor.

Tip: Build up your reps by splitting them into manageable sets of 15-20 reps at a time and adding on more sets with a short rest in between as your strength develops.

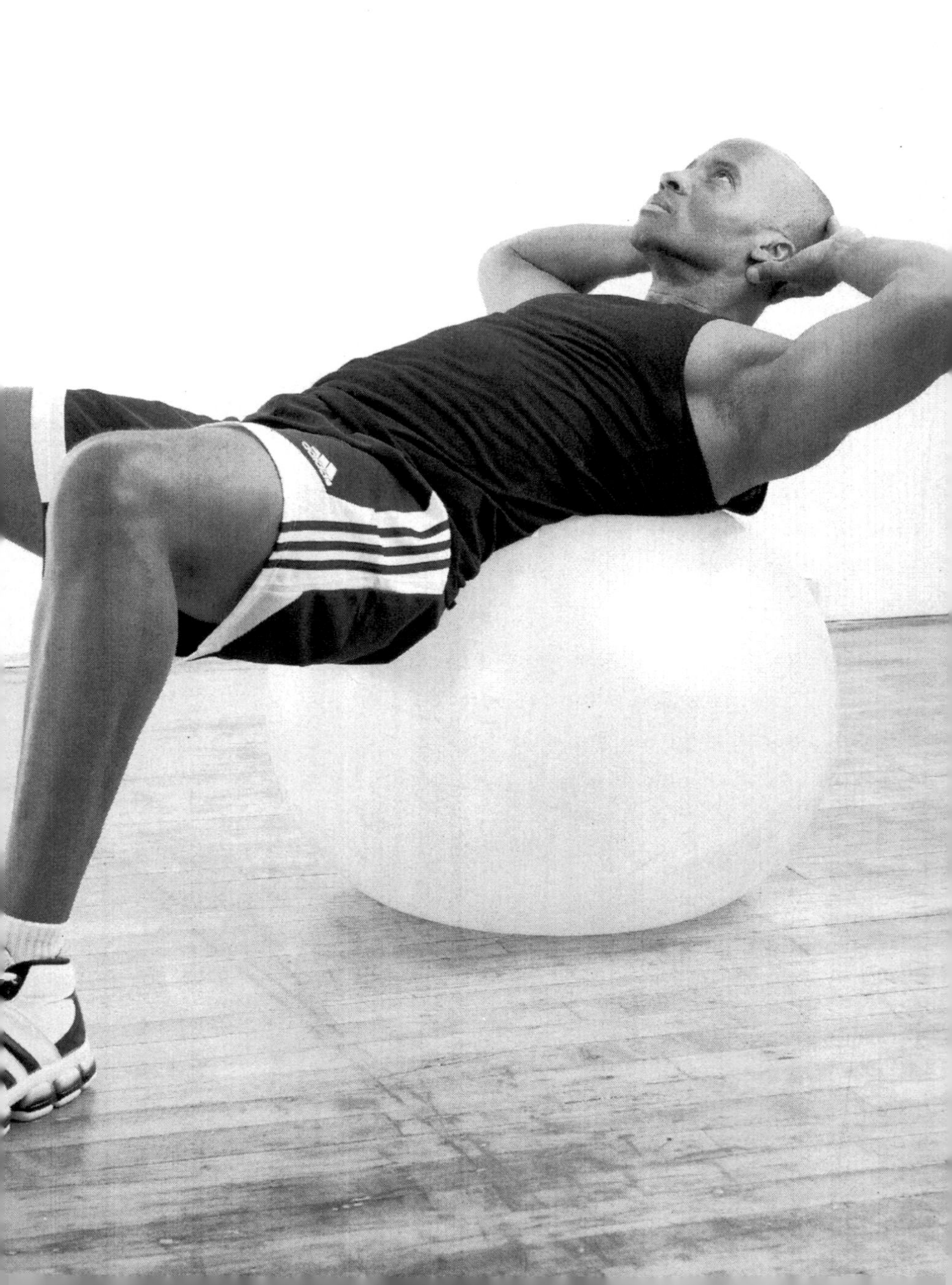

Too Cute to Sweat Exercise 6
Dining Room or Kitchen Chair Dips

Equipment: All you need is a dining room or kitchen chair.
Target Area: The triceps muscles at the back of your upper arms and the front of your shoulders.
Exercise:
• Sit on the edge of a chair and position your hands beside you to grip the front edge of the seat.
• Slide your butt forward off the chair, leaving your hands in position gripping the front edge.
• Slowly lower your butt toward the floor by bending your elbows. Go as low as you comfortably can—without actually sitting on the floor. You may need to shuffle your feet forward on the floor to allow enough room between your butt and the edge of the chair to be able to do the dip.
• Use your arms to lift your butt back up to seat level by straightening your elbows, being careful to keep the joints relaxed.
• Repeat the dip without sitting on the chair.
Repetitions: Every time you go to your dining or kitchen table, do 25 chair dips. They are great for defining and toning your arms.

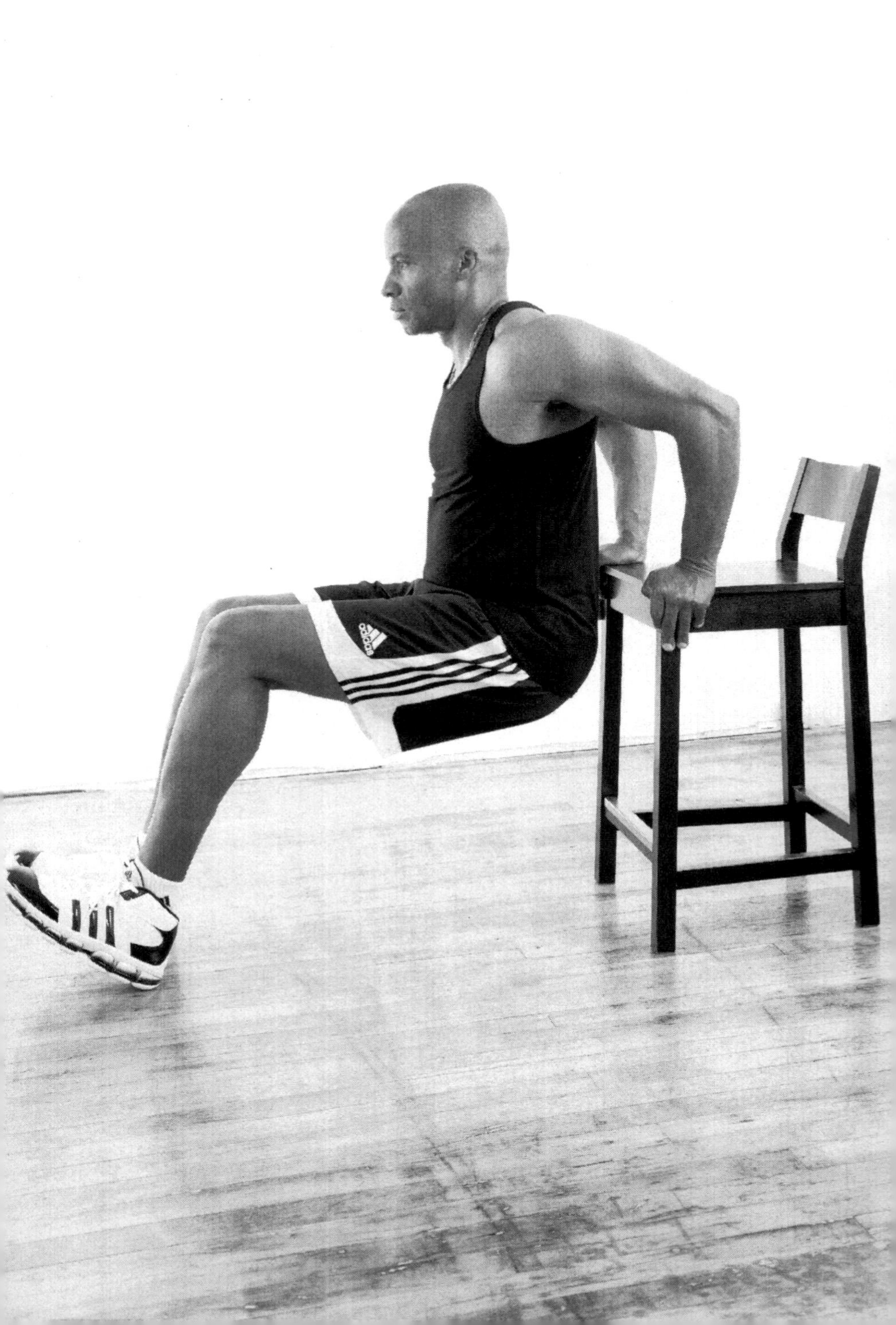
adidas

Too Cute to Sweat Exercise 7
Dining Room or Kitchen Chest Press

Equipment: All you need is a table or kitchen counter top.
Target Area: The triceps, chest and front of the shoulders
Exercise:

• Stand facing the table or counter and position your hands against the edge about shoulder width apart, palms downward.

• Move your feet back slightly so that you begin to support your weight on your arms.

• Keeping good posture and your spine in line with your legs, slowly lower your chest towards the table or counter by bending your elbows. Go as low as you comfortably can but even a couple of inches is great to get you started.

• Use your arms to push you back up to the starting position by straightening your elbows, keeping the joints relaxed at the end of the push, ready to repeat the exercise.

Repetitions: Every time you walk by a table or counter top, knock out 10-20 standing push-ups. This is a great way to build a stronger upper body and also develop nice strong arms.

Tip: The lower you are able to drop your chest toward the table and the further back you are able to position your feet, the more intense the exercise becomes.

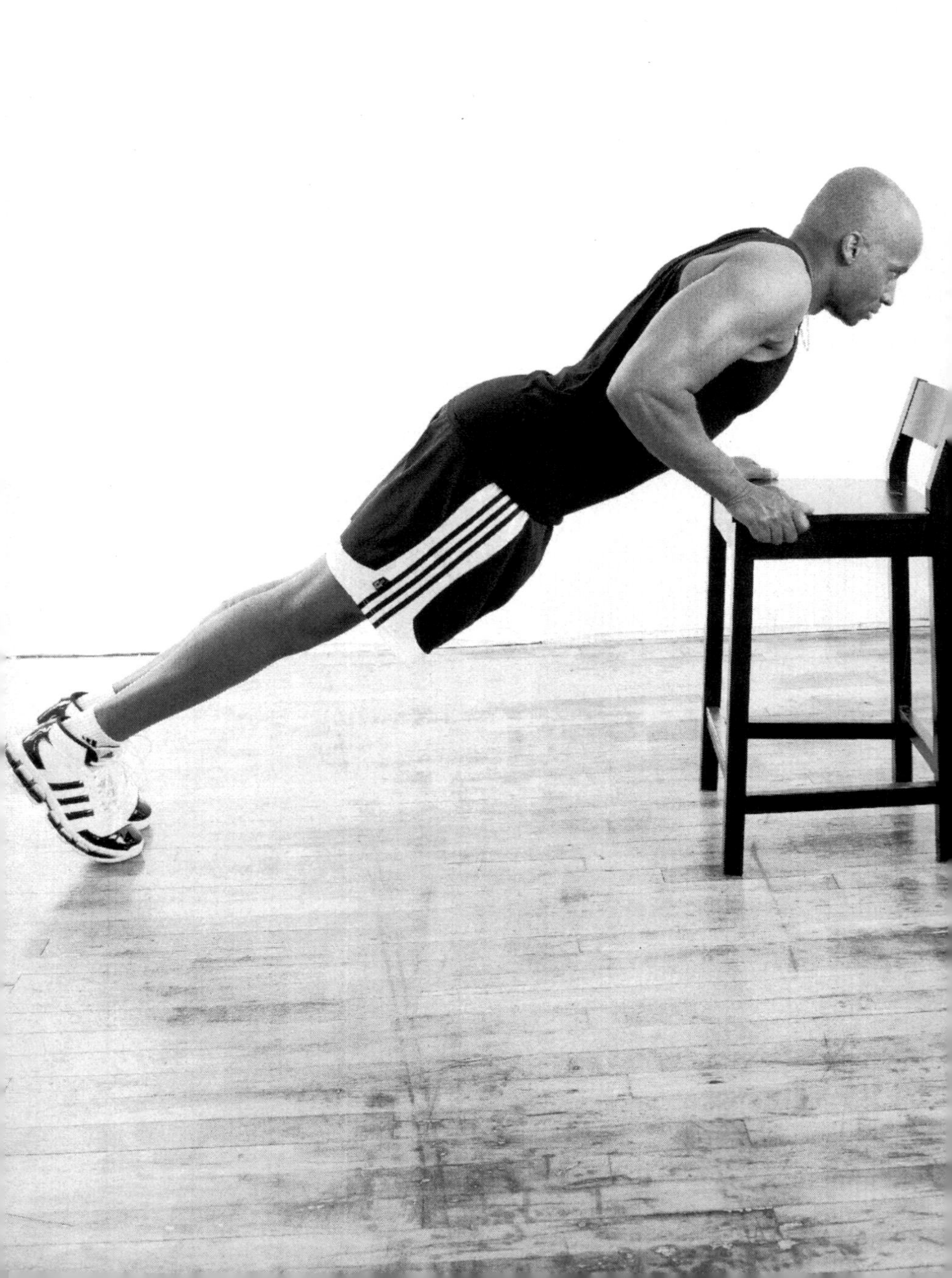

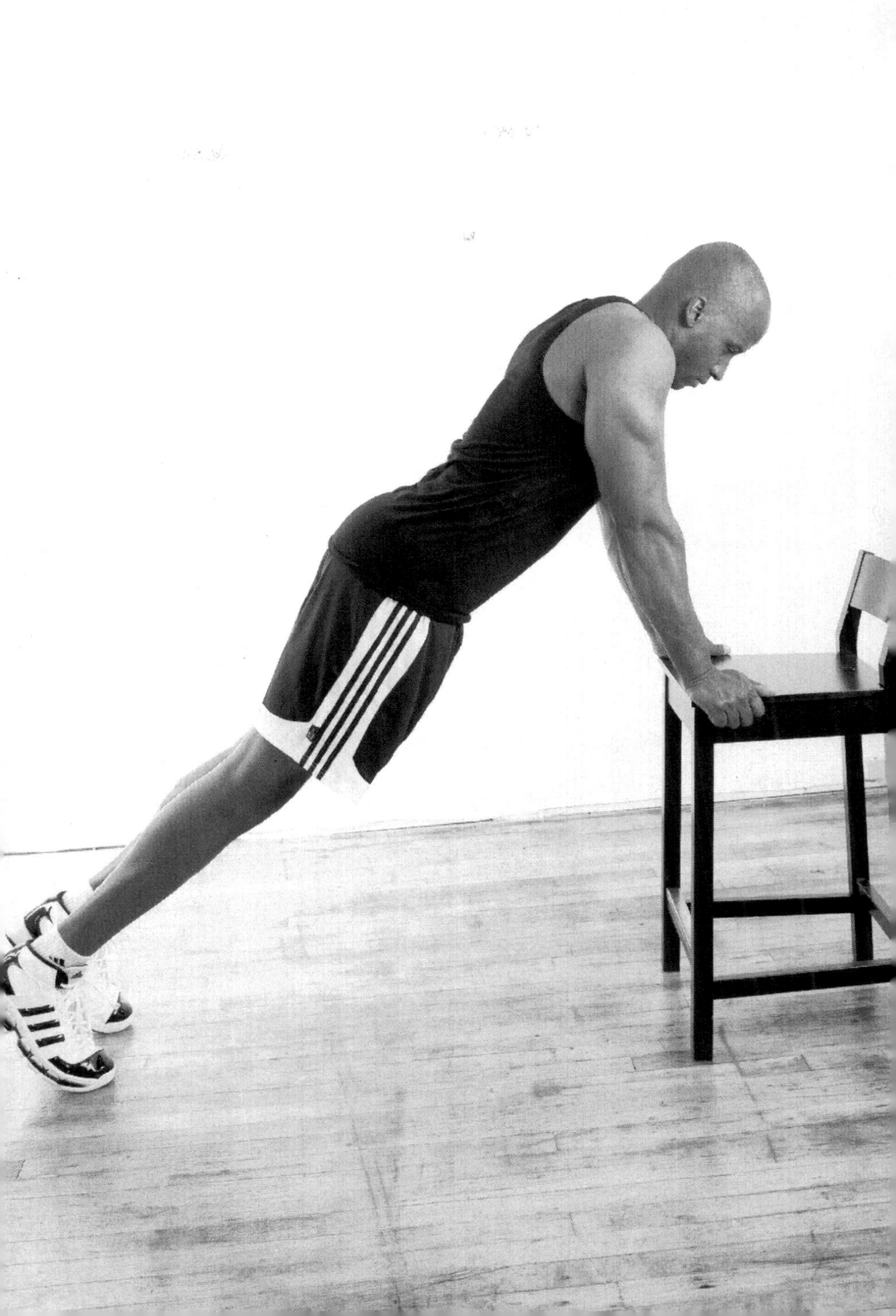

Too Cute to Sweat Exercise 8
Stairs Cardio Workout

Equipment: All you need is your staircase.
Target Area: Heart, lungs, and total body
Exercise:
Every time you go up and down your stairs, do 25 jumping jacks— so that is 25 jumping jacks when you reach the top and another 25 jumping jacks when you reach the bottom. If you go up and down your stairs 20 times a day, you will have done 500 jumping jacks in a day. Now that's a GREAT cardio workout.
Jumping Jacks:
The start position is standing with your feet together and your arms by your sides. The next position is feet apart and arms outstretched above your head so that you form a star shape. It becomes a jumping jack when you spring on your toes to 'jump' from one position to the next. From the star position, jump back to the starting position and then repeat the exercise to keep jumping!

Tip: If high impact exercises are problematic for you, you can try half jacks instead. From the starting position, take your right leg out to the side as you raise your right arm then return to the starting position to take your left leg out as you raise your left arm.

Too Cute to Sweat Exercise 9
Bathroom Dead Lifts

Equipment: A pair of 5-10 pounds weights.
Target Area: Legs and glutes
Exercise:
Use the weights that you already have in place in the bathroom.
• Squat down to pick up the weights from the floor.
• Stand up, holding a weight in each hand, keeping good posture in your upper body.
• Bend down, as if trying to touch your shoe strings, allowing the weights to almost touch the floor, and then stand up again.
• It's important to keep your back 'flat' as you bend down and lift, avoid rounding your back as you bend down or arching your back as you stand up.
Repetitions: Aim to do 15 repetitions and build up to completing three sets of 15 reps with a short rest between sets.

Tip: You can do dead lifts in conjunction with the Bathroom Shoulder Press.

Too Cute to Sweat Exercise 10
Bathroom Calf Rises

Equipment: No equipment is needed.
Target Area: Calf muscles
Exercise:
While brushing your teeth in the morning, lift up-and-down on your toes.

• Raise yourself up on to your toes and hold that position for at least two seconds.
• Slowly lower yourself back down but stop midway without letting your heels touch the floor.
• Repeat the exercise by raising yourself up again from the midway position.
Repetitions: Aim to complete 50 repetitions while you are brushing your teeth and build up to completing two sets of 50 reps.

What's Next?

It is okay to alternate some of these exercise moves to add variety to your workout and it is not necessary to do all 10 exercise moves in one day. The key is to do as many of these movements as possible as consistently as you can. You should never feel overwhelmed because this routine can and should be done within your daily lifestyle. After your 21 days, these movements will become a habit and you will be motivated to take fitness to the next level. Feel free to increase the amount of repetitions or weights to make the workout more challenging. The beauty of this program is that it is time efficient and effective. Remember, throughout the 21 day routine, drink plenty of water and take steps to minimize some of the unhealthy habits in your diet that you know are not good for you. Be sure to consume more fresh fruits and vegetables. Also, use a juicer to liquefy your fruits and vegetables when possible. Juicers can be found in a variety of stores, such as Wal-Mart or Target, at an affordable price.

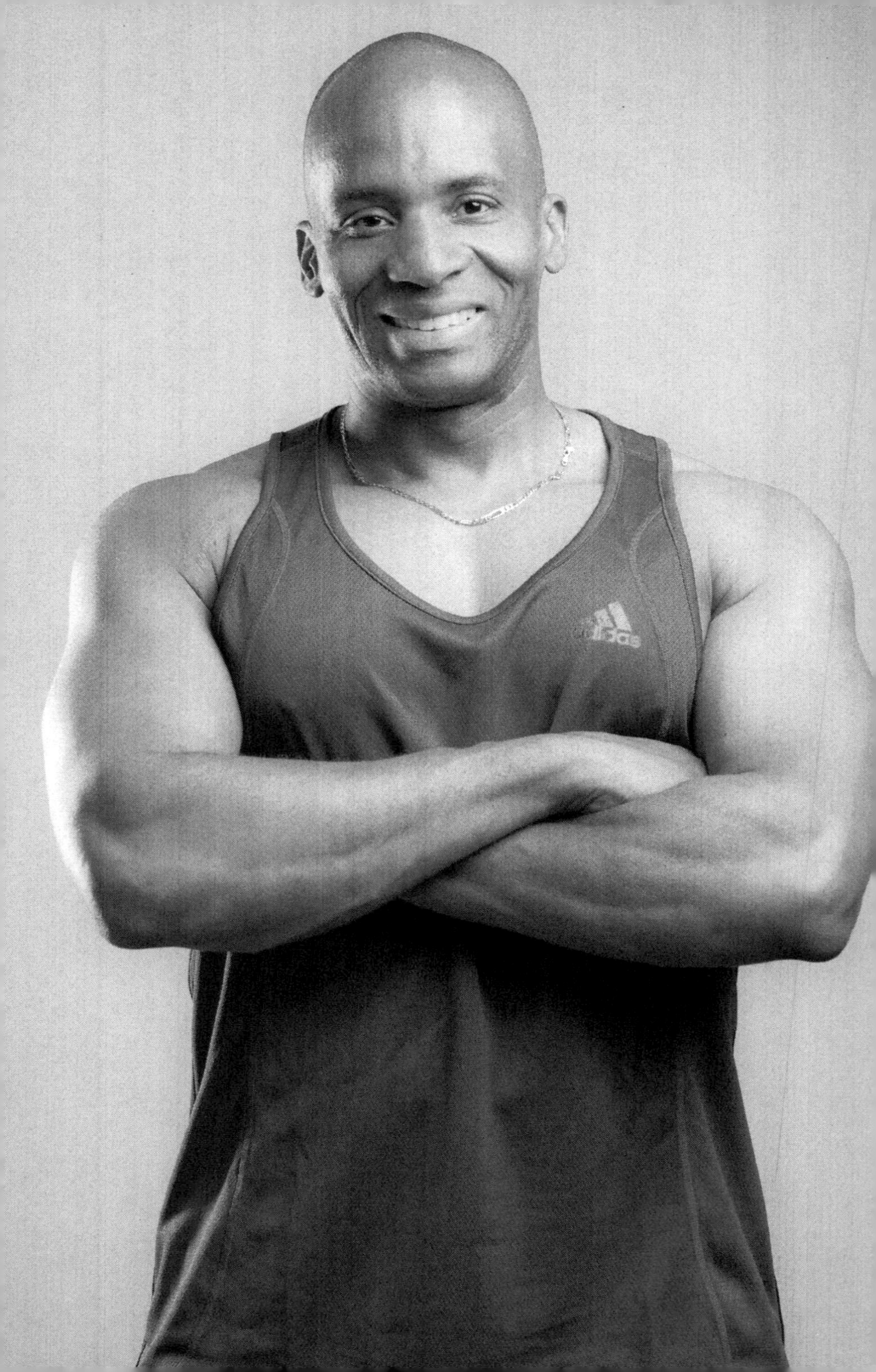

Chapter 11

Three Women Who Did It!

Beverly Richardson – 56
Married Mother and Grandmother, Career Woman and Student
Profession: Director of Development

How long did it take to start feeling good about exercise again?
I started to hit my stride and feel better after the fifth day. I would wake up a half hour earlier to do some of the exercises before going to work. Also, I incorporated some of the exercises between school studies. I would take a break away from the books and instead of running to the kitchen to get a snack I would perform some of the exercises.

Did you have any challenges to overcome during the program?
During the 21 days I had some personal challenges with some deaths in my family as well as a birthday; this didn't deter me from getting my workouts in. Exercise served as a stress reliever. Before starting the program I was not working out at all. This program was a great way to get me moving and taking care of myself again. Also, it made me more conscious of how to eat.

With your busy schedule, how were you able to get it all in?
I utilized my ankle weights the most in the program. I noticed mid-

way through the program that my clothes started feeling looser. I could tell that my body was getting firm especially in my lower extremities. Working out in my home was comfortable for me; it made getting in shape easy and convenient. Even after completing the 21 day program I still feel the need to work out and keep the program going, so now working out has become a healthy habit and is something that I look forward to.

What advice can you give a person who is starting this program?
Life can bring many challenges, but despite that you can still find the time to make exercise not only doable but fun. There is no place like home, use it!

Anastachia Thomas - 34
Married Mother of Two
Profession: Certified Licensed Day Care Provider

How were you able to implement the 21 day program having a home based business?
I incorporated the 21 day plan between the hours of 6am-6pm while I ran my day care. The program motivated me to go to the gym and exercise in the evenings. Being home for most of the day, the 21 day program was a good way to keep me active and energized which helped me keep up with my day care kids.

Was it difficult staying consistent during the program?
There were times I didn't really feel like exercising but I would feel guilty because the weights would be staring at me. I am a person who already enjoys exercise so I used this as a maintenance program before I hit the

gym at night. My favorite pastime is cooking exotic meals for my family and the kitchen was the place where I would do most of the exercises. I used the island in the kitchen to do push-ups and dips.

Did you see any immediate changes within the first couple of weeks?
I noticed my legs and arms started to be more toned and stronger very fast. My desire was not to gain muscle but to sculpt and increase my lean muscle mass.

Did you become bored with doing the same exercises every day?
Every other day I would challenge myself by increasing the weights and adding more repetitions. I didn't find it difficult or boring to finish the entire 21 days. I also stuck with the program even after completing the first 21 days. It's so enjoyable and I love the results.

Laila Saghir - 36
Profession: Registered Dental Hygienist

How did you feel about the Too Cute to Sweat 21 Day Fitness Program?
I enjoyed being able to incorporate the program into my already established daily routine. It was very easy to follow since none of the exercises were complicated. The instructions are user friendly, even for someone who is just beginning to exercise.

Was it easy to implement into your lifestyle?
Since I work full-time and don't spend too much time at home, I sometimes felt as if I did not do enough. I was not able to do all the exercises every day but I tried to complete as many as possible. On some days, I brought the resistance band with me to work and used it in my

lunch break. I was surprised to discover that if I really tried, I could find time to do some of these exercises even if I was not at home.

Did you feel as if the program was of benefit to you during your hip-injury?

Yes, I injured my hip running and my doctor advised me not to participate in any high-impact work outs in order to let my hip heal for at least two weeks. I was able to work on my upper body without adding pressure to my hip. I like the flexibility and the range of exercises the program provides.

What was the most enjoyable part of the experience and why?

The most enjoyable part was the knowledge that even if I did not go to the gym on a certain day, I still did something beneficial for my body and my health. In the beginning, I thought exercising in the bathroom was strange, but, the Bathroom Shoulder Press actually became my favorite exercise! I think I was most consistent with this exercise since the weights were always there and impossible to ignore.

Did you have any challenges?

My main challenge was remembering to wear my ankle weights. Since I am usually in a rush, I would sometimes forget to put them on.

Did you feel guilty if you missed a day of the program?

I never went a whole day without exercising, but there were certainly days where I could have been more productive. On such days, I did feel guilty about not completing more exercises but this was usually on days where I had already worked out at the gym.

What advice would you give to someone who is looking to get fit?

I would like to add that I have no doubt that this program is highly suitable for women who are unable to join a gym. It is all about being consistent and getting the job done. Results arrive from dedication and persistence and the great thing about this program is that it is designed to work around you, not vice versa.

Before I go, I hope you enjoyed this journey with me but, before I go I would like to introduce you to one of my favorite clients and friends. Sharon Page is a former Flight Attendant, Co-Author and Writer for Sister2Sister Magazine. As a Diamond President for Ardyss International, she has taught thousands of women around the world how to "Create Wealth While Promoting Health." Page is a powerful Coach, Speaker and Trainer with a mission to educate women on the importance of maintaining a healthy lifestyle. Her new book "Eat Your Food Naked" is getting rave reviews. Here is a excerpt!

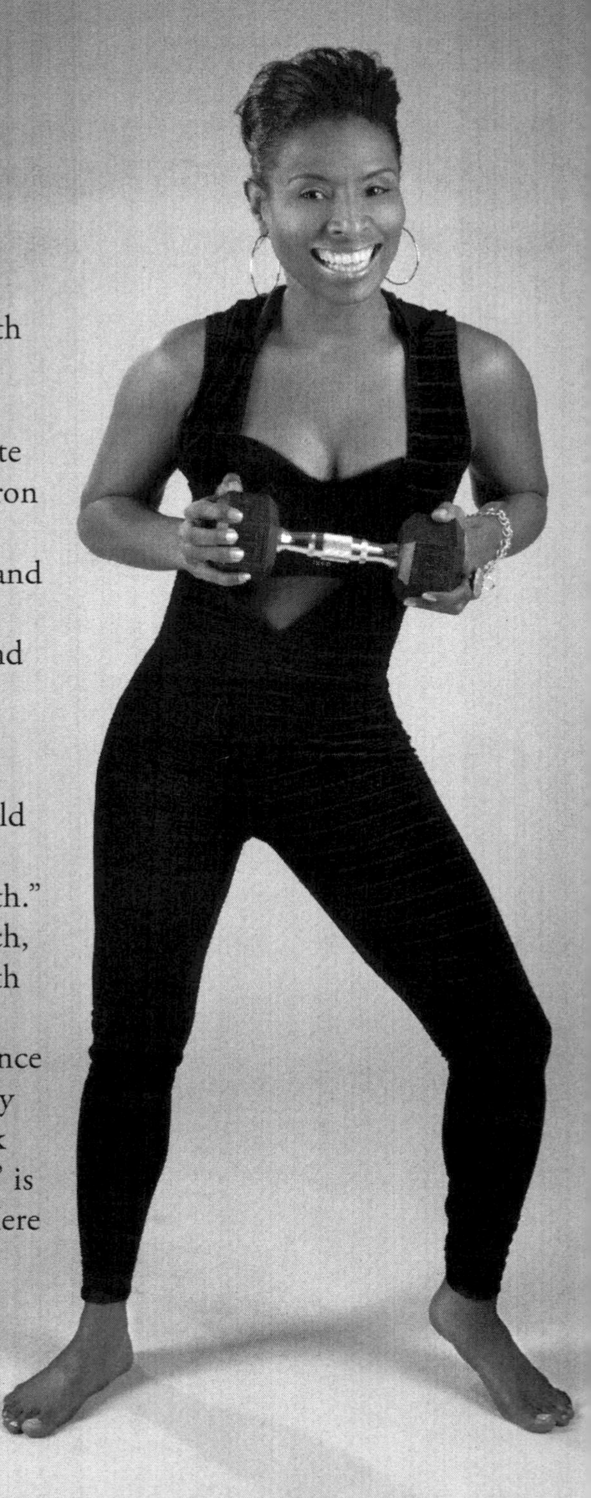

Real Estate

In my 30s, I was a Real Estate Agent. When it comes to a woman's body, I look at it as a piece of Real Estate. Real Estate is a valuable asset. It's personal property. Do you believe that your body is a valuable asset? It's God's temple, right? As a piece of real estate, your ultimate goal is to come off of the market, correct? Come on, ladies; you know that your ultimate desire is to use your sex appeal to attract Mr. Right to at least do a walk-through of the property (dating), that leads to a contract (engagement), and then go to settlement (marriage), and live happily ever after!

Notice that I said we use our physical attraction to "attract" Mr. Right. I did not say we use our physical attraction to go out and find Mr. Right. I said we use our physical attraction to "attract" Mr. Right. That's right, ladies, you should not be out looking for a man. The Bible says, "Ye that finds a wife finds a good thing." Not, "Ye that finds a husband . . ." That tells me that the husband is supposed to find his wife, not vice versa. But that's a subject for another book. Let me get back to my point. Okay, as I was saying, your body is a piece of real estate. Let me walk you through the process.

If your body is a piece of real estate, then that means it's a valuable asset. A buyer comes along (Mr. Right) and likes what he sees. The next thing he does is put a contract on the property (he asks you to be his girl). Afterward, he starts securing the financing, and, in the midst, he's observing his investment. He's checking out how much you eat, how much you make, if you work out, etc. You see, he's evaluating his ROI (Return On Investment). I don't know any investor who's going to invest in anything that will not appreciate in value—do you?

The next thing that happens is the "home inspection." This is the point where the buyer checks out the roof, the electrical system, and last but not least, he checks out the pipes and the plumbing. It's up to you to decide if you'll have your plumbing inspected before closing. I would "highly" advise against it! (smile)

Then, there is the appraisal. This is when the bank confirms that the property is worth the asking price. If the property does not appraise, the bank will not fund the transaction and the property cannot go to settlement.

> If you were a piece of Real Estate, would you make it to settlement?

There are reasons other than the appraisal that some pieces of real estate never make it to closing. One of the main reasons is, like many of us, many properties cannot pass the "home inspection." We don't take care of ourselves, or our bodies, so we have become that undervalued, dilapidated piece of Real Estate.

Take the test. If you were a piece of Real Estate—would you make it to settlement? Or would you be put back on the market because your roof is leaking (your weave is bad); you have electrical problems (you have no energy), or your plumbing is stopped up (you haven't been to the bathroom in a week because of your poor diet and nutrition). Do you know anybody who really wants to invest in a piece of dilapidated property? Start today to increase your own property value. Take pride in yourself. Make yourself a piece of Prime Real Estate. Go through your own home inspection. What's your appraised value? Are you worth your asking price?

It's time for you to make a decision to increase your property value so that you can go to closing and not end up like millions of undervalued real estate today—in foreclosure. I know you can do it......... I'll see you at settlement!